Editor *in* Chic

How to Style and Be Your Most Empowered Self

Mikki Taylor

ATRIA BOOKS

New York   London   Toronto   Sydney   New Delhi

ATRIA
BOOKS

An Imprint of Simon & Schuster, Inc.
1230 Avenue of the Americas
New York, NY 10020

First Atria Books hardcover edition May 2018

ATRIA BOOKS and colophon are trademarks of Simon & Schuster, Inc.

For information about special discounts for bulk purchases, please contact Simon & Schuster Special Sales at 1-866-506-1949 or business@simonandschuster.com.

The Simon & Schuster Speakers Bureau can bring authors to your live event. For more information or to book an event contact the Simon & Schuster Speakers Bureau at 1-866-248-3049 or visit our website at www.simonspeakers.com.

Manufactured in the United States of America

10 9 8 7 6 5 4 3 2 1

Library of Congress Cataloging-in-Publication Data

Names: Taylor, Mikki, author.
Title: Editor in chic : how to style and be your most empowered self / Mikki Taylor.
Description: First Atria Books hardcover edition. | New York : Atria Books, 2018. | Includes bibliographical references and index.
Identifiers: LCCN 2017040892 (print) | LCCN 2017051612 (ebook) | ISBN 9781501111716 (ebook) | ISBN 9781501111518 (hardcover) | ISBN 9781501111525 (paperback)
Subjects: LCSH: Beauty, Personal. | Women--Health and hygiene. | Fashion. | Cosmetics. | BISAC: HEALTH & FITNESS / Beauty & Grooming. | HEALTH & FITNESS / General. | DESIGN / Fashion.
Classification: LCC RA778 (ebook) | LCC RA778 .T3644 2018 (print) | DDC 646.7/2--dc23
LC record available at https://lccn.loc.gov/2017040892

ISBN 978-1-5011-1151-8

ISBN 978-1-5011-1171-6 (ebook)

To Mommy, who taught me how to live an empowered life,
and my Darling Husband and loving family,
with whom it means everything

Contents

Introduction *xiii*

1   Eye on Beauty *1*

2   Skin: It's a New Day *79*

3   Makeup: No Limits! *123*

4   Hands, Nails, and Footnotes *159*

5   Hair: Running the Show *183*

6   Style: Make a Statement *229*

7   Master You Inc. *271*

Acknowledgments *279*

Life is the perfection of a point of view
and a divine plan in action.

~ꙥ

Introduction

Wherever you are in the journey, this is your time to show up and style out! I've learned that the good life we desire begins within and is based on an appreciation of who we are, and impacts everything about us—from our fashion and beauty choices to the élan with which you live. Before you work that amazing lipstick or dream frock, I want you to be inspired by the Queen that *you* are and live with authority! Life isn't a dress rehearsal: this is it and it's about *living* your narrative from an empowered perspective—one that affirms you every step of the way. It's centered in valuing your truth and confirming that you are more than willing to embrace the cost as well as the delight of being your best self. It cost those who came before you. They not only had to make sacrifices for the future you now own, but had to make strategic choices, both personal and political, and so do you. It costs something to be your best self and it's called determination. It costs something to stay on course—commitment—and for certain, it'll cost you to own your life to the fullest. What I know for sure is living with vision comes down to making the purpose-driven choices that support you and your desire to live the life you want *now*, not the one you're waiting for. We don't have the time or the luxury to live two lives. There's no better time than right now to express yourself boldly and define what's truly important to you.

So take that essential inventory on everything: your dress code, your life code, your love code, who you surround yourself with—in short, how well you're authentically living your life, because your behavior must testify that you know who you are! The goal is to see where the person you envision yourself to be is at odds with the life that you're carrying out. Before you decide not to do the work, or think it'd be too overwhelming, ask yourself this pivotal question: Is it a challenge or an opportunity to be your most empowered self? Know that whatever area you babysit won't grow, so push for the possibilities! Real style is all about living your truth, and you must be willing to live on purpose in order to thrive. Know that it takes decisive and prayerful work to thrive, not just survive, so see it through.

I've come to know that you must have a relationship with your decisions and not make them on the fly. I've been guilty of doing the latter, and it always cost me in ways that threw me off track and kept me longer than I wanted to stay. Now I take my time because I know the only way I'm going to be disciplined enough to see my decisions through is by being clear and fully engaged with them from the start. The Word says, "Where your treasure is, there your heart will be also," so each of us has to decide what's important in life so our hearts will stay focused.

For certain, faith must be a part of your strategy. Faith is nothing if it's not defining your life. Faith is what keeps you going when you'd rather resist. It's what anchors your "soul's seat" and keeps you steady in rocky times. Some of the most visionary women I know are conditioned to prevail by a transformational faith that's real in their lives. As such, they're strategic, fully committed gals who stand on God's promises and rock! I admire how they continually activate their dreams and walk in their purpose because they have a clear understanding that "faith without works is dead," as the New Testament says. When you possess an unshakeable faith, you can move through life with a keen understanding of who you are, no matter what, because you believe what God says about you to be true, and that's a winning strategy for sure!

I know the importance of not just looking together but *being* together and loving the journey. I've worked with and met some of the most fascinating people in history, and what it taught me for certain is this: if you're not owning your truth, then you're only living in the shadow of who you are meant to be. Real women stand firm; are resilient in the face of adversity; honor their strengths; nonjudgmentally address their weaknesses, ups, and downs; and possess a fearless, unshakable sense of self. I'm so passionate about this that I've gathered some of the most powerful women I know from all corridors—from the arts and entertainment industries to corporate America and more—to have their say on what compels them to stand in their truth and what fuels their self-appreciation, purpose, and strength.

I penned *Editor in Chic* because I want every woman to own her life and master her distinction with the kind of panache that sustains her in every way imaginable. Thirty-plus years in the editor's chair as beauty and cover director of *Essence* magazine has me full of information and yet all the while passionate about new and noteworthy ideas, so whatever your beauty and style concerns, whether it's how to navigate your look at any given time and determine the most fab practices or how to define a bankable wardrobe that's truly you, I've simplified the process with inspiring ideas on these pages. Like you, I love it when someone comes to the table with the kind of solution-oriented information that works in my day-to-day, so whether you're standing in front of the mirror trying to figure out a great "five-minute face" or wondering how to pick the most sensuous lingerie (that also supports your assets!), I've got you covered.

I need to tell you that Ms. Mikki loves a steal, so I'll show you how to be frugal and look fabulous (some of the best beauty picks can be found in the drugstore, and chances are that dress you're drooling over can be found at a reduced price online) and where to invest your time (e.g., renewal practices—a massage, a luxurious bath, a meditation session) and money (customized hair color, a timeless LBD [little black dress], professional skin care services) and more.

EIC also shares motivating insights on mastering "Brand You"—what you stand for—and establishing a platform that showcases that divine-inspired purpose that lies inside of you with great success. Each of us must identify and master our purpose. Purpose is that unique talent, that is to say that gift that you stand in possession of and the compelling requirement that is placed on your life by your Creator. It's no wonder it burns inside of you like a dream that must be awakened! In fact, the New Testament urges you to "stir up the gift that is in you," and if you look back at your childhood, you'll see the clues to your purpose. For Yours Truly, it was about playing with my dolls and telling stories, which I did until age fourteen. This led to a career of creativity with living dolls and my life's work to affirm and inspire millions of us on the pages of *Essence* magazine. It also compelled me to empower beauty companies to carve out effective marketing initiatives, messaging, and products that resonated with the magazine's audience of "beauty enthusiasts." Today I'm continuing the work as editor-at-large, and fulfilling my mission of affirming us through engagements that do just that. I'm speaking to the media and across the nation at conferences and colleges to women of all ages on beauty, empowerment, and spirituality, and empowering future generations through the Disney Dreamers Academy with Steve Harvey and *Essence*, to ensure that none of us live beneath the richness of who we are. In short, wherever Mikki Taylor is, you can rest assured that "purpose is at work."

When it comes to defining your purpose, one thing is certain: you must ignore the voice of reason to uncover and thrive in it. When I came of age, they weren't asking little brown girls like me if we wanted to be editors. They put limited choices before us, but I didn't choose any of them! My mother taught me that to be risk-averse is to be success-averse. What I say to you is this: your purpose may not have an established title or path, it may not make sense to anyone but you and God, but that's validation enough, so don't let anyone or anything stop you. Conquer your fears and move forward by faith and put the divine plan in action, and you will succeed.

It is upon all of us who are privileged to walk in the dreams of our ancestors to pursue excellence and use our gifts to make a difference because the world is waiting to receive what God has placed in you. That is what purpose at work is all about. In the grand gesture of things, it is purpose that orders your life, directs your actions, and brands your future. And no matter where you are on your dreamscape, you must recognize that you're the entrepreneur of your destiny and you must be transformational in your thinking, fearless in your ambitions, and determined to succeed in your purpose.

I'm a big believer that opportunity favors the prepared mind. Those who are not only willing to do the work but also work their divine plan with strategic intention always *command* their goals. I've found the ease lies not only in focusing your energies and overcoming procrastination, but also in surrounding yourself with what I call a "celebration circle," a circle of celebrants who are there for you no matter what the season of your life. Your greatness was not designed to work in isolation, so don't move through life unsupported. Life is challenging enough as it is, and you need a team of empowered people whose support you can count on, who are test-worthy and there for you no matter what you are going through. Make no mistake about it: it is about connecting with those who want to see you win. I know I couldn't do without my council, and I don't want you to be without one either, because it's practices like these and others found in *EIC* that will help you succeed.

EIC also offers an entry to meet every purpose in your life and quotes to fuel your soul and inspire you along the way. There are blank pages to hold your notations on the all-important self-discoveries you'll make and, believe me, these personal insights, inspirations, and affirmations are empowering to your journey. Because my name is on it, *EIC* not only shares what works, but also reveals *what* and *who* doesn't, from toxic people dressed up as "friends" (because I don't want you hallucinating, thinking that they've got your back when they're really invading your life and trespassing your value) to the products that overpromise and underdeliver (that's called "imposter marketing"!).

At the end of the day, I want you, as Queen & CEO of You Inc., to be informed, inspired, and fearless! To paraphrase Oprah, who, after hearing Viola Davis's acceptance of her 2015 Emmy, tweeted, this is your "proud to spell your name W.O.M.A.N." time! So get your imagination in gear, redefine what it means to be a leading woman, push for the possibilities, explore new options, and set your mind for success so you can engage the affirming life you deserve. Power to your journey!

Mikki Taylor

"There can be no happiness if the things we believe in are different from the things we do."

—Freya Stark, explorer, travel writer

1

Eye on Beauty

I love taking in an afternoon at the Metropolitan Museum of Art's Costume Institute on New York's Museum Mile. For Yours Truly, the most electric exhibitions are those where I can don a headset and learn about the inner workings of the showcase I'm about to see. Before we talk *beauty* and that which the outside world takes in about you and me, let's talk about the inner template, that which directs the external showcase, because if that's not in place, then nothing else I speak of on these pages really matters. I don't care for "smoke and mirrors" and never really fell for hocus-pocus. I like substance, that which is so provocative its unique value is clear and downright compelling. Translation: empowered women who know who they are live boldly, and their appreciation of their authentic selves is so clear it's nonnegotiable! Now let's talk beauty.

AFFIRMATION

"I am fearfully and wonderfully made."

—Psalm 139:14

If the Creator thought His vision of you was so masterful that He created only one like you, then you'd better give evidence that you know how amazing you are!

Mikki-ism

POWER POINT

If your inner coach isn't affirming how fierce you are, fire her!

Own the Queen in you: "Good Morning, Queen, let's kick off this day in celebration of the unique, divine-inspired woman that you are and all that the King has masterfully done in creating you! You will not need to seek validation today. The King has already validated you and fully empowered you to be all that He has designed you to be, so go out and rule!"

Imagine if this were how your every day began, in celebration of all that you are, with gratitude and full assurance that you are more than how you look, what others think of you, and even the beliefs that you allow to get in the way of the truth. It would certainly redirect your outlook, let alone some of the things you allow to compromise your way and disempower you. The Creator says when He designed you and me, He was satisfied, but our complaints and lack of appreciation of our uniqueness convey that at times we feel differently. Without question, it's so important to take pride in being your authentic self and appreciate all that you are. And yet, as much as that might seem like a given, we are often our own taskmasters. We complain about the things we don't like about our bodies. We negate our beauty or compare ours to that of others we consider amazing. We push ourselves beyond reasonable limits, trying to prove that we can do it all. We jump through the hoops others have set up for us in life and in the workplace, hoping coffee will take us up and a glass of wine will calm us down at the end of the day, and we regard much-needed "time for self" as selfish rather than one of life's nurturing luxuries that lies within our power. Practices like these and others shut out our much-deserved time to edify our spirits, restore our temples, and explore the life we each desire. Every gal has a list of things that get in the way of her honoring herself and owning her life as the rich and rewarding experience it is meant to be. So much of our life's experiences are programmed and in sync with the ways of others that we've become adept at living life "on demand." The challenge here is if you're not careful, everyone will have the remote control but you! And what's happening is empowered women are becoming disempowered by training themselves to become adept at doing more while running on less. The catch-22 is their life's priorities are now falling on a never-ending wish list. Some dolls don't even have time to be tired anymore: they've got that on hold, too. It doesn't mean we're not doing well—we look good on LinkedIn, Instagram, and Facebook. It just means our well-being is at stake. That's an unfair trade policy! Been there and I'm not repeating the class. I decided quite some time ago to become wholly engaged in my life and stop passing through it. I made restorative "time for self" a priority because only then could I serve with an open heart and not resent missing out on what is essentially renewal time, something we all need. You see, resentment over any lack—real or perceived—will cost you and it will always keep you longer than you want to stay. Moreover, it robs your inner and outer beauty and deletes your peace. I say it's time to press reset and own the Queen in you and decisively do what it takes to thrive because true Queens serve by example and how well we honor ourselves shows that we acknowledge our worth. It also says that we understand our relationship and value to the King. Author, inspirational speaker, and host of OWN TV's *Iyanla: Fix My Life* Iyanla Vanzant reasons, "The only way for the Queen to rule effectively in her life and in the 'kingdom' is for her to have a loving, intimate relationship with the Source of her life and her power." Knowing who you are and whose you are is critical as it has a direct impact on how you treat yourself as well as how you'll allow yourself to be treated. As a Queen, you can't settle for mediocrity in your thinking or in your actions because the King wants the best for you and He has equipped you to discern it in abundance. This is the kind of awareness that will keep your beauty, your temple, and your emotional and spiritual well-being together. It's what empowers you to keep your thoughts positive and your self-esteem on high as it reminds you that you have been created in a serious image and a divine light, and nothing and no one can overshadow that. Therefore, you must understand that in order to wear the crown effectively and remain in command, you must be balanced and affirmed and make the time to step away, refuel your spirit, and nurture your temple. Doing so doesn't call for a destination vacation, though that's nice. Sometimes it calls for a staycation, a day of peace and solitude, an hour of no technology, a time to commune with your Creator. In short, be discerning enough to administer to yourself! When I was growing up, my family didn't take vacations as we know them today. My mother and my father were entrepreneurs in Brick City, so we took car trips, day trips, or a holiday weekend. So the notion of a long vacation is still somewhat foreign to me as it wasn't modeled for me in my formative years, but I know quite clearly that I must take a mental and physical break, if for no other reason than, to paraphrase the old adage, "all work and no play makes Jane a dull gal!" On a more serious note, it's essential to my body, mind, and spirit, and that's reason enough for me to engage in those practices that nurture all three.

Don't become adept at doing more while running on less. Press reset!

Mikki-ism

Wake-Up Call

Many of us use an alarm clock to get up on time in the morning and start our day. I say why not take a moment and use this time to set the tone for your day? As part of my morning meditation, I decide what I'm going to bring to my day by selecting a power term(s) and setting this directive in motion, and all day long this promise serves as a reminder, no matter what. Remember, the power of your thoughts can either move you forward or hold you back. Here are a few of my favorite terms of inspiration:

- Purpose
- Determination
- Focus!
- Patience
- Resilience
- Gratitude
- Defy expectations!
- Work excellence
- You got this!
- Have a great day!

Quality Control

Devote one workout per week to your mind. Be it yoga, tai chi, or a guided meditation, practices like these create awareness, focus on breath work, and give the mind a chance to connect to the body and help you to relax, harness stress, and stay balanced. Resources abound for you to practice these mental and physical disciplines, whether in the privacy of your own home or in the formality of a class, so why not give them a try? Remember, any form of introspection is a valuable opportunity for renewal. Don't miss out: make time for yourself and label it a priority.

The ability to master life and be all that you are destined to be is inextricably bound to how rich you are when it comes to the "inner me." This calls for continuous introspection, assessment, and exportation of those things you can't use. You can't put away what you won't identify, and there's no time like the present to rule with an intentional vision. On the surface level, when you show up fine and fierce, you make God look good. When you are overwhelmed, depleted, full of erroneous guilt, and high on complaints and insecurities, you misrepresent. The King didn't purpose you and me for that. He created us to be the praise of His glory, and we must honor that which will enable us to be at our best. According to Vanzant and other experts, in order to reign in full, you must possess the vision to do so. "A Queen's vision is what will keep her grounded and focused, less reactionary and more responsive, and cause her to live every moment purposefully, prayerfully, and playfully," says Vanzant. It also fuels your discipline, commitment, and determination, all essential to your inner beauty. So decide today that you're going to get used to doing what it takes to own the Queen in you.

66 "There is no passion to be found in playing small—in settling for a life that is less than the one you are capable of living."

—Nelson Mandela, anti-apartheid revolutionary, former president of South Africa, Nobel Peace Prize winner, legend

Be Inspired

I learned early on that life is only as good as you feel in it, which is why I bring joy with me wherever I go. Trust me, more than anything found in a jar, it's what really helps you to get your glow on! It's my driver, and I find it in the little things, like how a chic red lipstick works my full brown lips. I find it in the moving moments of high-fiving a sister on how fierce she is and in the awesome experience of an answered prayer (so I keep my "Amens" ready). I even find it in the midst of a "pity party" by having a good laugh at myself when I realize that I might as well quit this experience as nobody's joining it but me! Hands down, I find it in the soul of the woman who looks back at me in the mirror. When it comes to your inner beauty, perspective is everything. It's what determines how you both regard and outwardly express the Queen who lives within.

Don't follow where you should lead!

Mikki-ism

I had an inspiring role model for my script in my mother, as she was the kind of gal who appreciated herself across the board and as a result filled her size-nine shoes in every way imaginable. She celebrated each day with a clear sense of purpose from her predawn prayer time to her sophisticated style sensibility (pressed jeans, matching shoes, and bags); from her many award-winning coiffures to how and when she took her meals, where she shopped, how she traveled (monogrammed suitcases in tow), her work ethic, even her relationships. She was choosy and passionate about living an inspired life. She was a real visionary thinker who taught me that attitude is everything, as this is what makes all the difference in how you see yourself and how well you'll make the kind of distinctive choices that support who you are.

Noticeably, my mother's world was filled with like-minded gals who were *self*-inspired and lived with great joy and gratitude no matter what life served at the table. Women like the legendary Ella Fitzgerald, who brought her signature flair to everything she did, from her perfect pitch and unerring sense of timing to her chic short cuts, even her fabulous fold-out Xmas cards that my mother always hung on the mantel during the holidays. Never mind her great battle with diabetes or the racism she faced when on tour, it didn't steal her joy or cause her to devalue herself or shrink from her divine purpose. Another doll who comes to mind is the stunning singer and pianist Carmen McRae, whose powerful sense of self, enchanting eyes, and captivating style both on and off camera always fascinated me yet never conveyed her share of emotional ups and downs in the business. And then there was the American icon that was Sarah Vaughan. My mother and Sarah became friends during their school days, and later, when Sarah wanted to try out at the Apollo Theater on Amateur Night, my mother got together with a group of friends and they put together the money for Sarah to go and try out as her father didn't want her to sing secular music and so didn't approve. Talk about a challenge! The rest, as they say, is history, and today we have her gift, as well as the many dazzling album covers my mother directed of this chocolate beauty who soared in a nation at a time when those of us who looked like her couldn't even sit in a restaurant alongside some of those who loved her music. Talk about an inspiration—she would be most amused today at being the subject for a US postage stamp! I loved learning how empowered Sarah was in spite of racial prejudice and so many other "behind the scenes" stories from my mother because they were not only exemplary of the way she lived, but also taught me that life isn't perfect: it's what *you* make of it that counts. What also stuck with me was learning that when Sarah became "the Divine One," as she was known, she bought the house we lived in across the street from hers in the heart of Newark, New Jersey, so my mother could be close. She engaged my mother as her everywoman—secretary, hairstylist, makeup artist, and wardrobe stylist—and together they traveled the world. When you know who you are, you surround yourself with the right people as you recognize those who believe in you, and their gifts complement yours.

Later, when my mother retired from the road, she opened her own hair salon in Newark's Central Ward, serving award-winning looks to women from all walks of life. This for me was essentially "beauty school," in that I got to really observe all types of women who lived their lives from an inspired perspective. Take my aunt Laura, for example, who was one of my mother's devoted clients. I didn't realize until years later that she was "the help," in that she did "days' work," as it was referred to back in the day, keeping house for a white family at their main residence as well as their summer home in Cape Cod. I only knew she was away most of the time, and her only day off was Thursday, which I lived for. That was the day when she'd pick me up after school for dinner, dressed to perfection in the perfect frock, complete with pressed white gloves from Germany, coiffed hair, and a barrage of etiquette lessons for Yours Truly to practice while she cooked and told stories. I loved listening to the way she spoke, pronouncing each and every word with great diction, and watching her flash that fabulous gap of hers in a smile that made me proud to be her audience. Ditto for the way she raised a perfectly manicured brow to emphasize a point or two as opposed to dropping an expletive! Believe me, she took great joy in that! Truth be told, if Aunt Laura or any of the women in my mother's life didn't own their joy and weren't inspired from within to set the tone for their lives, I might see things differently today. They were all glamorous, lived the life they created, and money or the lack thereof didn't dictate that or compromise it. They defined that from a supreme sense of self-awareness and pushed past their challenges to embrace the possibilities. Oftentimes, we stand in the way of our own joy and sabotage our ability to thrive without even recognizing it. According to Dr. Nicole LaBeach, master life and relationships coach, who has a coaching practice in Atlanta, Georgia, we must be intentional about our joy and stop being so focused on what's feasible and what can happen. "The heart has a song, but we have found a way to tone down the volume or shut it off," she says. LaBeach compares this state of mind to high blood pressure: the heart starts to struggle to pump blood to itself, and it begins to develop a buildup that blocks the arteries, and "it's not until you stop the clogging of the arteries that you can smile." Research has proven that when the heart is healthy, everything else has the ability to flow. The same holds true for your internal perception and the inspiration that you derive in setting the tone for your life. So ask yourself, "What brings *me* joy?" Not your girlfriend. "How inspired am I by the Queen that lies in *me*? What breathes life into her soul?" Be honest with yourself so your heart can thrive and your joy will become so powerful that it's infectious!

The power to live inspired lies within each of us, and we owe it to ourselves to use it. At the end of the day each of us must realize that life is a gift and how we possess it is up to us. Susan L. Taylor, *Essence* editor-in-chief emeritus, founder of National CARES Mentoring Movement, and a woman who's forever dear to my heart, taught me that we must learn to enjoy the process of life—all of it. In so doing, we each have the power to create our own narrative and carry it out with joy and determination.

AFFIRMATION

"Life loves to be taken by the lapel and told:
'I'm with you, kid. Let's go.' "

—Dr. Maya Angelou, poet, author

_____ Inspirations . . .

A Decisive Moment with Author and Civil Rights Activist James Baldwin

It's quite magnetic when someone lives his life in such a way that he pro-
vokes joy in others. I remember the late James Baldwin, the legendary poet,
essayist, and novelist, was a lot like that. He had what the French call that
joie de vivre, a real zest for life. I met him back in the '80s when he came to
the *Essence* offices for a visit, and I was immediately swept away. It was joy at
work in the brilliance of his conversation and in the magic of his laugh, and
it infused every room where he was present. Baldwin had the kind of spirit
that inspired you to do something greater than you could imagine and to
boldly ask yourself, "Why not?" This grandson of a slave and Depression-era
child, whose genius took him from Harlem to Paris, living in the most complicated of times, talked of simplicity and sincerity of purpose. He spoke to the
work those of us at the magazine were privileged to do and what it meant,
and mentally I rose several levels that day. I don't think I came to *work* a single day after that experience, but rather I came to serve and recognized the
joy in doing so. Whenever I think of him, a smile curls at my lips because he
made me realize that joy, well, it's such a simple thing, but it has the capacity
to make a tremendous difference in your life and the lives of everyone you
touch. Every day that you live, remember joy is a choice, so don't let negativity get in your way. It's a roadblock that costs you time and energy, and you
can't use it. Be reminded that your joy can only be altered by the things you
allow to have control over you and your perspective. Every time someone or
something presents itself in a way that threatens to compromise your joy or
redefine your truth, refute it. Affirm this in its place: "The Creator wants me
to live an abundant life, not one that's impeded by the negative energy of

others or the obstacles that seemingly come to defeat me and steal my joy."
Be inspired to own your joy and bring it along for the ride wherever you go!

AFFIRMATION
"As he thinketh in his heart, so is he . . ."
—Proverbs 23:7

You need to learn how to lovingly accept compliments because folks are really bragging on God, your architect, when they compliment you!

Mikki-ism

_____ Inspirations . . .

In the Moment with Jill Scott, Singer, Songwriter, Poet, and Actress, on the influence of empowered women, being your authentic self, and living full throttle

"I allow myself to be myself because I think the alternative makes you ill. Pretending all day is so exhausting. . . . So I say live, honey, full potential."

"I'm an only child, and growing up, I loved it. I appreciated my alone time, and as a writer I would find places to be away from everybody to discover the things I loved about myself. Once you find the one thing you love about yourself, you find more things and they become important. I've been inspired by so many women in my life, women like my grandmother, who shaped a lot of who I am. She had style (she would even get dressed up to go to the doctor!) and grace and a sweet loving spirit. I saw her in love as a child; I saw her strengths. One time she ran into a burning house to save her child, and she fought off all these men to do so, and though she came out with her eyebrows and her eyelashes gone, she did it. She lost her husband and was left with five children to raise, and people said, 'I'll take this one and I'll take that one,' and she said no. Then there's my list of egots: Whoopi Goldberg and Barbara Streisand, plus Bette Midler and Diana Ross, my creative muses. They're renaissance women, they're actors, singers, they're multidimensional, and they inspire me. I have amazon women in my family, all the women are five foot nine and up, they're all ample, big-bosomed, and very shapely, and they inspire me. Every flower in the garden is different, and you have to acknowledge your flower. Yes, you're going to change, you're going to get a pimple or a pouch that you keep or lose, that's life, but you have to have the stuff on the inside that empowers you. Some people may not get you and that's fantastic, not everybody is meant to be your friend, not everyone is meant to understand you, not everybody is going to get it, but you have to continue to forgive them 'for they know not what they do.' I don't see what benefit it is to wish to be someone else when you've been blessed to be yourself. Be that. I'm a big fan of spa days, and making my own lotions, and burning essential oils in my house. I'm a wanderer, and finding places where I can disappear is integral and it keeps me balanced. So I find places where I'm just Joyce's daughter. I think all of that lifts me from the inside. It doesn't matter how much makeup somebody puts on me or what kind of hair hat I'm wearing at the moment. If I'm not at peace, then I'm not beautiful to myself, no matter what anybody else sees. I prefer to be beautiful to myself. We're all in the same boat, and we're going through very similar things all the time. I think that's what drives me. I have this deep longing, burning, impatient hunger, to lift people, and my intention is to give them permission to be human because sometimes people need to be human, to just be! To be reminded, you're good. If you want to cry right now, baby, have at it. I probably will join you. If you want to go on a vacation by yourself and experience quiet, have at it. I want to see us grow, I want to see us love, I want to see us have these feelings and get back up and *allow*. I have stage fright and I have to battle it every day. I allow myself to be terrified—I don't talk myself out of being terrified—I talk myself into moving through it. Sometimes I have to sit down and take fifteen breaths and remember who I am and who God is—it just is what it is. That's part of living, but I know that I can't allow fear to rule me. I allow myself to be myself because I think the alternative makes you ill. Pretending all day is so exhausting. So I say live, honey, full potential. I have a friend who was killed and Kim was always accused of being beautiful and she would say, 'Oooh, you should see my insides, if you think I'm beautiful, that's great, but if you could just see my insides.' And I always remember that. If you could just see my insides, be beautiful on the inside. That's what really matters."

Know Your Value

How do you see yourself? Your life should demonstrate that you know who you are. Heaven rejoiced the day you were born, for you were composed under divine inspection and signed, sealed, and delivered by the hand of Him who framed the wonders of the universe and you are His chief creation on earth. The King in validating you gave you a set of truths in your Genesis statement: not hashtags but truths, one-of-a-kind, divine-inspired, *unprecedented*! Nothing like you ever was nor ever will be again, so know who you are and don't let anything in life, or anyone for that matter, eclipse or diminish your "it-ness" as a Queen. Take care, too, that you don't allow any opposing standard to infiltrate, compromise, or devalue your worth—do so by setting your boundaries. This must be your nonnegotiable platform. "Self-perception is the key to every success, every victory, every joy-filled moment, and every heartache or heartbreak," says a woman whose hard work and life experiences are a testimony of what it means to know your worth, Iyanla Vanzant. Your view of who you are has a direct influence on you—personally, emotionally, and professionally—so you must possess a distinct "value-acknowledgment factor" about yourself. Research has shown that we tend to act in harmony with what we perceive ourselves to be, and the read here is this: you're not going to love yourself and live any better than what you believe to be true, so you've got to be clear as your perspective establishes the tone for *everything*. You should challenge anything that you have stamped yourself with that isn't in agreement. In her practice, LaBeach instructs women on the importance of properly evaluating the template of how they view themselves. "God created us in a view that was pretty intentional," she notes, "and the further our self-view moves away from how He sees us, the more we struggle." You do yourself a great disservice when you don't recognize who you are, and you make it easy for others to define you, and that's too much power for anyone to have over your life. The King didn't empower you only to have you become disempowered by others. Vanzant cites "learning to stop looking for, searching for, expecting, and requiring external validation" as one of her principal lessons. When you know your value, you won't waste your time auditioning for others' approval and reinventing yourself so they'll like you. Instead, it'll compel you to reinforce yourself and stop going where you're tolerated and go where you're celebrated. You don't have any business being around people who don't understand and appreciate your value. Get off that bus—that's not your stop!

66 We must reject not only the stereotypes that others hold of us, but also the stereotypes that we hold of ourselves."

—Shirley Chisholm, educator, author, first African American and Democratic Party candidate to bid for president of the United States

Your self-esteem should be so on point, you wake up every day excited to be you!

cMikki-ism

_____ Inspirations . . .

In the Moment with Marjorie Harvey, CEO of The Lady Loves Couture, Wife of Entertainer Steve Harvey, on self-appreciation and staying centered

"I'm empowered because of my belief in God and knowing He doesn't make mistakes. He made me in His image—what is there to doubt?"

"When I was growing up, I learned 'if God said it, that settles it.' People can put all kinds of stipulations on your life, but if God says I'm great and I can do all things through Him, that's it, and I don't have to wonder. Steve and I talked about this a while back and acknowledged that people are always going to talk and paint a picture of who you are, but nobody can do that better than you—that's 'coming straight from the horse's mouth,' as they say. I'm not afraid to say I've messed up, of failure, because they are much better teachers than getting it right all the time. No one gets it right all the time. Knowing who I am, believing in myself and my family, and prayer keeps me centered. Prayer is at the heart of who I am and how I manage my life every day. I've also found if you don't verse yourself in negativity, which is toxic, you don't have to worry. You also have to study the Word, there's no other way around it, and be in the presence of good teachers. Better to have what you need in advance. My grandmother used to say, 'Get to know God before you need Him because the hour of need is not the time to make introductions!' In your hour of need, you want to be on a first-name basis with Him because you've been talking all along."

When I'm out and about, people always ask who's my favorite among the many celebrities and personalities I know and have worked with. The truth is, I have many, but names aside, the women I admire are those who live from the inside out, as opposed to the outside in; from my observation, one is secure and the other is completely shallow, often unstable, and far too easily swayed by circumstances and the opinions of others. This is not the definition of knowing your value and being engaged with the truth of who you are. It's never about what's taking place outside of you; it's about what's taking place within you. It's not even about status, for that matter, because positions come and go and your self-view must be about more than your title experience. I've worked with empowered women from all walks of life and career corridors—the corporate world, arts and entertainment, politics, including First Lady Michelle Obama—and my admiration is huge for any gal who can fill her own heels and not wobble! I say this because life, people, circumstances, and more will test you to see what you're made of, and that's what separates the real women from the girls in training. Real women stand firm, are resilient in the face of adversity, honor their strengths, nonjudgmentally address their weaknesses and ups and downs, and possess a fearless, unshakable sense of self. At the end of the day, what they all have in common is the ability to be strong, secure spirits, utterly aware and in full control of who they are, and that makes them simply the best. Here's the last word on what fuels a sense of purpose, strength, and self-appreciation from some empowered women I know:

66 I keep at the center of my mind the great gift/demonstration Madiba gave us all. You can't always control circumstances, but you do control your response to those circumstances. The true power we all possess that no one can contain, constrict, or usurp is the power over our own thought."

—Alfre Woodard, actress, producer, political activist

"We should all know our value as we navigate our lives through this world that we live in. It is necessary now more than ever. What fuels my sense of purpose is seeing how hard my Haitian mother worked to get us into this country so that I could have the opportunities that I've been able to have. That makes me walk with gratitude, and it gives me the strength to continue. And I appreciate that strength because as women we are so strong. No matter what the challenges are, we rise above them."

—Garcelle Beauvais, actress

"What fuels my sense of purpose and strength are my mentors, mentees, and the youth who are working hard to change the world for the better. When I see myself in other people and am motivated and pushed by them, I learn to love myself more and more. Strong Black women are my backbone."

—Misty Copeland, first African American female
principal dancer in the American Ballet Theatre

"I am truly honored to be a Black Woman! In the spirit of my mother and my grandmother, I am dedicated to carrying out the Principles instilled in me of respect, hope, and most importantly love in the way I live my life, in the joy of serving others, and in our children, to whom the future belongs."

—Pauletta Washington, singer, mother,
wife of Academy Award–winning actor Denzel Washington

"I believe in me because God believes in me. The Word says, 'I am beautifully and wonderfully made,' and I don't allow anyone to tell me otherwise."

—Cookie Johnson, author, philanthropist, founder of CJ by
Cookie Johnson, wife of NBA legend Earvin "Magic" Johnson

66 I believe God loves me and has a plan for my life. I'm grateful every day for the people and situations He brings in my life to manifest my purpose, starting with the most loving mom and dad I could have ever dreamed of."

—Michelle Ebanks, president of Essence Communications Inc.

66 To know your value, you need to know yourself. Trust yourself, trust your instincts. We all wonder if we are smart enough, good enough, talented enough, pretty enough—whatever the words are that we put up in front of ourselves. You've got to work to get rid of that and it's not easy. It's a constant struggle back and forth, but every time you come up against it, you've got to say, 'Why not me?'"

—Cheryl Boone Isaacs, former president of the Academy of Motion Picture Arts and Sciences

66 One of the blessings of growing older is being able to see with greater clarity the urgency of leaving a legacy of having lived your beliefs. Upon reflection, I saw that there was little sustained progress and advancement for people of color and women representing talent in the entertainment industry. Talent, even when they were vocal advocates for their own hiring, didn't seem to connect the dots and realize that to *not* see themselves reflected in the faces of people they hired signaled to the industry that they didn't appreciate their own value. Ultimately, what gave me the courage to speak up on this issue in forums that might perceive my message as being against their self-interest was realizing my own value and appreciating that my self-confidence fueled my success, and I could turn that belief in myself to the advantage of others. Demanding that people in my industry with the power to hire be truly empowered by empowering others was a turning point for me and affirmed my belief

that we all have the ability to make change happen, even in the face of entrenched customs and practices."

—Nina L. Shaw, entertainment attorney, founding
partner at Del Shaw Moonves Tanaka Finkelstein & Lezcano

66 We have all been blessed to enter this world with a gift and promise of having purpose and destiny in our lives. With this promise, it empowers me to know that my value has already been predetermined by God. It's my responsibility to follow a path that allows me to achieve my purpose—walking in the light, enduring faith, and doing the work to make the world a better place."

—Mattie McFadden-Lawson, founder and president
of the MML Design Group

66 I know that after a few decades on this earth that my purpose is to use the very best of who I am to invest in other people to inspire, motivate, and help them to be their very best selves and to maximize their success. I am also clear that you must embrace and appreciate all of who you are, wherever you are in life, if you want to reap the opportunity to advance, improve, and get to your next best self!"

—Carla Harris, American gospel singer, author, and vice
chairman, wealth management, senior client adviser,
and managing director at Morgan Stanley

66 People often say, 'Failure is not an option,' but failure is reality. You will fail at some things in life. The question is, can you learn from your mistakes, can you push through failure to succeed? That's growth, that's development! I live by the motto 'A setback is nothing but a setup for a comeback!' It's served me well!"

—Michelle Miller Morial, mother, wife, journalist

66 **M**y grandparents Dovie and Frank Jackson raised me with the Biblical notion that God rewards truth, hard work, and service to others. I was told that God would honor me with a rewarding life if I would keep to those tenants. I must say that having that foundation and attempting to adhere to those teachings (even on days when I was not so successful) continues to provide me with a complexity of confidence, power, courage, wisdom, charity, and peace. I have been blessed with a fulfilling life with family and friends, and I am grateful every day for the opportunity to navigate this incredible, maddening world. I seek God in all things."

—LaTanya Richardson Jackson, actress, philanthropist,
wife of actor and film producer Samuel L. Jackson

66 **I** truly believe that God has a purpose for everyone's life, although some people will never venture to find out exactly what that purpose is. My purpose was placed in my lap like a neatly folded napkin, and as I fought to regain my normal life, it was very clear to me that life was done. When my sun/son was shot and killed, I was so broken, and in my mind I never imagined that I would ever be happy or smile again, but God had other plans for me. Please know that even during my brokenness, I told God thank you because deep down inside I knew that someday He would give me the strength to get back up. I stood up when my son was shot down. Look up and you, too, will stand up."

—Sybrina Fulton, founder of the Trayvon Martin Foundation

66 **T**here is no force equal to a woman determined to rise."

—W. E. B. Du Bois, author, historian, civil rights activist

Knowing your value also means having the capacity to teach people how to treat you, and it's not always about what you say but what you do. In other words, how you carry yourself. I remember working with "the First Lady of Civil Rights," the awe-inspiring Rosa Parks, on a shoot for the 1993 *Essence* Awards, when she, along with Lena Horne, Aretha Franklin, community activist Sweet Alice Harris, and several others, was being honored. I was so in awe of her quiet strength and the dignity with which she carried herself, and I could see how she overcame white supremacy just by her refusal to allow herself to be treated without the respect *she* knew she was due. Her self-view and her nonviolent act gave birth to the civil rights movement and the Supreme Court's decision to declare segregation on buses unconstitutional! That still speaks volumes to me. To this day, I feel the same about the late Dr. Betty Shabazz, a role model for millions of women, who, widowed in her twenties by the hand of assassins, persevered to raise six daughters, earn a doctorate, and then pour the truth into the lives of others as an educator extraordinaire at Medgar Evers College in Brooklyn. I came of age in full knowledge of the tragedy that had shaken her life, and when I had the opportunity to meet her in 1992, I was beyond inspired. Her spirit bore no burdens, nor anger at the past. She was joy on "full" and had a smile that made you feel as if you'd known her for a long time. She, too, possessed a dignity and elegance that made you sit up straight and long to be in her company, knowing that you would be blessed there. The world stood still in my heart the day she passed.

The New Testament says that "the older [seasoned, mature] women should teach the younger women to be reverent in the way they live," and I can say I've learned from the best. They've taught me about carriage, dignity, and the value of making the right response as opposed to reacting when others don't do the right thing. The purpose is to maintain your poise. As Michelle Obama so eloquently put it at the 2016 Democratic Convention, "When they go low, we go high," and I think this is a life mantra for empowered women. The Queen in you must execute self-control in order to not misuse your energies or forfeit your dignity. Even in your day-to-day, don't allow yourself to be played by reacting to minor stuff with major attention. It's not worth compromising your value just to meet someone on their level of behavior and sacrifice yours in the process. Leave that to the reality-show divas and soap stars that are getting paid to show out.

> Shallow things only define who you are and increase your attractiveness to shallow people. Don't take the bait!
>
> *Mikki-ism*

Finally, you must learn to make a distinction between feedback and criticism. "There are times when people give us feedback, information that we can use to be better or do better the next time," Vanzant says. There are also times when your detractors will criticize you out of envy and because you are comfortable in your skin, and you must recognize the difference. If what is being said doesn't hold up against the truth, it has to be dismissed, no matter where it's coming from. You cannot be at peace if you are not centered in an identity that transcends the judgments of others or the circumstances that life brings your way. When you put your faith in the right place, you don't have to worry about either. I say don't let your human nature be a roadblock to your spiritual nature. Our natural instinct is to lash back when someone hurts us, because that nature is weak, but don't play chess with your emotions by rendering evil for evil. The Word tells us "love is not easily provoked." It takes spiritual maturity to know how to handle criticism in a way that doesn't offend in return by taking on dysfunctional behavior. On a deeper level, your self-worth and your value-acknowledgment factor are part of your power, and there's no sense having that power if you don't get it; don't let others know you have it, and your opponents know Godly wisdom dictates your restraint! Enough said.

Do know that self-acceptance is a powerful motivator. Refuse to conform to standards that have nothing to do with you.

Mikki-ism

_____ Inspirations . . .

In the Moment with Beverly Bond, Founder of Black Girls Rock, on finding value in the valley, overcoming fear, and walking in your truth

"Every time you think things aren't going the way you want them to, that's a problem for you to solve. It identifies where you need to do the work, and that work is where you get to go to the next level."

"As a child, I didn't embrace physical beauty as much as I embraced inner beauty. My mother helped me appreciate my value, and in teaching me value, she helped me to appreciate life. She also made me aware of appreciating the beauty of life as a child of God and being truthful to myself by doing the things that honored my calling. I was an introvert, but being an introvert does have its advantages—you answer to the beat of your own drum, and among the many lessons, you learn not to be a follower and to value your own thinking. What became my biggest confidence booster was discovering what I'm passionate about and being able to do the work that took me on a whole other level of success. It wasn't without its challenges, though, because when I started deejaying, I got thrust into the boys' club and found out that all the boys don't want you here. This was a level of sexism that I had never faced before, where guys were trying to diminish my presence and my value. Life is a growing process and we're all going to go through it, but I've learned there's value in the valley. Every time you think things aren't going the way you want them to, that's a problem for you to solve. It identifies where you need to do the work, and that work is where you get to go to the next level. What helped me to overcome my fears and pursue my dreams was immersing myself in a two-and-a-half-year program that helps you peel away the layers and live in your truth. I was looking at music as the ability to transform this festering, sexist culture and I had the expertise. When I came up with Black Girls Rock (because we know it!), initially it was an idea for a T-shirt. The plan was to write down all the names of the powerful women I could think of, from Harriet Tubman to Susan Taylor and more, and I ran out of paper! I said THIS is bigger than me and it's bigger than this T-shirt. This is the word we need to hear. I knew this platform was going to make a difference and cause us to see ourselves as beautiful as we are. I had to challenge the glam of the counter-message—not to knock the video girls, but I needed to show us in other ways. I wanted to create a space where Black girls could find a more holistic narrative of who we are. In addition, if you looked at mainstream media, we were absent or stereotyped, and in looking at movies we were hardly ever the love interest of our men. If you turned on the music on the radio, it didn't reflect what was going on in the street. It wasn't you and me connecting, it was how we as Black women performed in bed, so when you think something's by design, you have to design something else. I said I cannot accept that narrative that my Black is not beautiful, that we can't be leading ladies. I discovered that I have a voice and that *one* voice can make a difference. I love mentoring young women and seeing that they appreciate who they are and that they are learning to love the skin they're in. We all have to be very focused on finding our truth and walking in it."

66 **T**here's plenty of room in the world for mediocre men. There is no room for mediocre women."

—Madeleine Albright, first female Secretary of State

_____ **Inspirations** . . .

In the Moment with Sanaa Lathan, Actress, on self-nurturing, spiritual guidance, and perseverance

"You're doing great, keep your eyes on your own path."

"I've learned that you really have to take care of yourself and shore yourself up to run your own race, otherwise you'll go crazy. To me it's a constant balancing act and I made a commitment to myself. The first thing I do when I get up is meditate for twenty minutes. People say, 'I don't have time for this,' but you'll spend twenty minutes on the internet. It's really about prioritizing your time, and when I don't do this, I don't feel good. I give myself social media fasts because it lowers your vibration and in turn lowers everything around you. What you're seeing on social media isn't the truth. People are always presenting what they want you to see. It's like, 'Look at how amazing my life is.' I think this is important for everyone. When I first came to Hollywood, I had a spiritual guidance counselor. She was different than a life coach and I talked to her for ten years and I learned how to navigate as a healthy human being in Hollywood. I even credit her for getting me the role in *Love & Basketball*. They wanted a basketball player that they could teach to act. They kept looking at basketball players, but director Gina Prince-Bythewood couldn't get me out of her head. Finally, months after coming back in and rejecting me, I got the role. People in my family and my best friend said, 'This is wrong, drop out.' It really felt like I was being strung along. My spiritual guidance counselor said, 'Even if you don't get the job, this is a test of your faith, and instead of attaching this to the end results of getting the role, just go in and play it.' It was a struggle, but she kept leading me back to that mind-set. That shifted my thinking and I got the job. If I had dropped out, who knows where my career would have gone. I'm a storyteller and I was put on this earth to entertain people through my work and to have a huge impact on the culture; that is the intent and I feel very blessed. Every character is about what I'm trying to give to the world. I think it's important to step out of my comfort zone, to be a little scared and take risks. I'm always pushing myself, and through that comes a fulfillment and a joy. Looking back, if I were to write a note to my younger self, I would say, 'You're doing great, keep your eyes on your own path.' "

POWER POINT

An empowered woman knows that great style—the kind that has an impact not only on how you look but on your very presence— is a reflection of the critical work she does to master every aspect of who she is.

Saving Grace

In this digital age that we live in, where everyone speaks in sound bites and acts in an urgent "hit send" behavior concerning anything and everything, I think it's critical that we make it a point to operate with graciousness. You can't talk to me about style and what defines a woman without having graciousness in the mix as I just won't hear of it. To me, graciousness is really "conscious living from within," and it's an essential factor of being the change you want to see. Far more than good breeding and good taste, it really comes down to how you act and what you want to be known for. Here's my checklist on what defines a gracious woman:

- **Composed:** Cool, calm, collected, well mannered.
- **Inclusive:** Recognizes the value and worth of all people, aims for unity and acceptance.
- **Cooperative:** Able to work with others and make them feel at ease.
- **Compassionate:** Considerate, warm, openhearted, understanding.
- **Receptive:** Easy to converse with, open to possibilities.
- **Forgiving:** Allows room for error in herself and others.
- **Empowered:** On purpose, assured, operates from a position of strength and love.

Treasure Your Vision Space

Recognize that your mind is your command central and it's your duty to regard it as your most sacred territory, for it's the center from which you are able honor yourself and direct your actions. Everything in your life stems from how you think and what you'll accept as fact, as well as the falsities that you allow to take up space in your mind and compromise your style. In order to make sure the right messaging is centered there, take care with regard to what enters in and has the ability to influence you. Be sure you are nurturing what you want to grow and starving what you want to check. If you don't, you'll be easy prey to the traps of thinking that you aren't beautiful and can't work the fiercest makeup hues, execute your purpose, or slam anything that you are more than creative enough to do, because it's what's inside of you that has the power to motivate or defeat you. As Vanzant notes, we must guard against being assaulted by our own terroristic thoughts! When the wrong information is present, doubt and confusion will take over and you'll find yourself energizing your worries and investing in your stressors. Worse yet, you'll impose all kinds of limitations on yourself that will brand you as a "victim" and cause you to settle for less when you should be reaching for more! This is not who you were meant to be; this is not the directive that was predetermined by your Creator in your Genesis manual. The *Queen* that God created is equipped to walk in all her glory with full intention and dominate the stuff that comes against her. In this tech-paced, nearly haywire world, where we're evaluated from an ever-changing perspective, you must be the gatekeeper to your mind and not give an all-access pass to that which will short-circuit your assurance, insult your intelligence, and destroy your strategy to live your best life.

I became fascinated by the role of the point guard over the years in my work with the WNBA during Rookie Weekend and on tour visiting the various teams. It is the most specialized position in that the point guard has the big view of the game and essentially possesses and protects the ball so the team can score. Think about how crowded it gets on the court. Opposing team members are trying to seize the ball and break the strategy. There's noise from the stands, and fans and opponents alike are all having their say about the game. Now think about your sacred space. Life is a lot like the game itself, and how well you score has a lot to do with how well you guard your mind. Personally, I like being the point guard and keeping my eyes on the big picture, and there are days when I'm blocking access to my vision space so I can tap into my strengths and win. When I'm in preparation mode, it's about getting still and doing an all-important self-examination, recognizing any negative thoughts so I can release them. I don't want to be bound by useless stuff weighing down my clarity and creativity. This is what should motivate each of us to keep our "dwell time" in the truthful places, not in the negative spaces that don't affirm us.

Remember God's promises and rock!

Mikki-ism

In protecting our minds "we also must expand our emotional vocabulary beyond happy/sad, right/wrong, good/bad, and angry/okay," Vanzant says. The way I see it, if the Queen is going to secure her sacred space, she's going to need more "internal subjects" at her disposal than this handful of characters! Part of ruling effectively lies in recognizing that we're human, not perfect. "We make poor choices and bad decisions, but they are not fatal, nor are they a testimony to our essential being," Vanzant concludes. We all have days where we are less than our highest and best self and our internal conversations can shift like the wind. Don't trip it or camp out there. There's so much more to you than any one day, any one choice or decision. For that matter, don't dwell on the past. There's very little that any of us can do to reach back and change it. Some of us are tormented by events and circumstances that happened in the past and we refuse to let go. Why sacrifice your peace? Take the wise path: If there's something you can do to change what's tormenting you about your "yesterdays," do it! If you need to forgive someone, act on it and stop fueling what has in effect become a burden for you. If you need to apologize to someone or right a relationship, do what's in your power and know that it is enough and let it go. Break the weight of the past so you can live fully in the present and affirm a clearer future. Above all, keep it moving, sis, with the determination to love yourself as fervently as God does and choose to *encourage* your spirit rather than be the taskmaster. Meanwhile, don't lose sight of your "human card." Only one is perfect, and that's God, so stay in your lane!

> 66 **R**emember no one can make you feel inferior without your consent."
> —Eleanor Roosevelt, former First Lady of the United States, diplomat, activist

Finally, don't be guilty of assessing your clout and what you can and can't do according to those who don't mean you well or in places where you are the invisible woman. Keeping it real, I'll be the first to tell you not to hit up a cosmetic counter that doesn't have foundation shades that speak to your beautiful brown skin or a retailer that excludes your dress size! Think about what that has the potential to do to your psyche, let alone what it says about the value of your business. I'm with LaBeach, who reminds us that the "thought" is the master of all other parts, so you have to manage it for your good.

_____ **Inspirations . . .**

In the Moment with Aja Naomi King, Actress, on inner beauty, mastering rejection, and getting still

"You have to cherish you and realize that you are an endangered species and appreciate your uniqueness. What a waste of that uniqueness if you don't!"

"When I was growing up, going to school wasn't super easy as we were the only Black family on the block and I was typically one of two African Americans in class *and* the only dark-skin one. I knew I was beautiful and smart because of my parents, who not only told me but who just loved up on me and my sisters. In life, there's a lot of outside noise and I have to quiet that and that inner critic that we all have and look at my truth, where I am and how far I've come, and embrace that knowledge and power inside of myself. I knew

I wanted to be an actress at the end of my junior year in high school, and I was willing to make the sacrifice to pursue this seemingly intangible dream, despite knowing that it might result in my being sad, alone, and hungry! I also knew that I would disappoint the expectations of others, but this was my life and I didn't want to regret not trying. The regret seemed like a worse burden to me than any other possible outcome. The toughest part is the constant, unending rejection. I realize that there's always going to be some work or campaign that you know in your heart that you are perfect for and would like the opportunity to show what can come out of you, and they'll say 'no.' That 'no' often feels like they're saying 'no' to everything that you are, and it's momentarily soul-destroying, but then you realize there's an opportunity out there for me and we are trying to find each other! That there is that thing that's going to come at the right time and you're ready for it. There's always going to be something negative coming at you, but we must realize that we all have the power inside of us to refute it. You have to cherish *you* and realize that you are an endangered species and appreciate your uniqueness. What a waste of that uniqueness if you don't! Diversity is still an issue, on screen, off screen, and in the offices where they make all the decisions about who's going to have these opportunities, but I'm inspired by women like Shonda Rhimes, Viola Davis, and Kerry Washington, who've become the masters of their own destiny. I even include myself in that—to be visible on a television screen or a movie screen and to know there's some girl out there who's inspired by seeing me. And I'm especially inspired when I think of those that will come after me and take it even further. I make it a point to take time with myself by getting quiet and having pure 'me time' to think about life and how I'm feeling. It's like a personal check-in from head to toe, and it helps me recognize that I need to let this go or pursue this other thing more or ask: Am I okay with everything around me and my current situation? I always come out of it feeling refreshed and renewed and with a more specific vision of what I need to do next. It's an act of self-love really, one that we all need to indulge in more."

66 I like our style. I like the fact that nothing gets us down for very long. I like the way we aren't afraid of trying anything once and good things twice. In a world that continually assaults all that we are and that we stand for, I like the fact that we have stood and are standing for ourselves."

—Nikki Giovanni, poet, writer, educator, activist

Truths like this are among the many reasons I loved being beauty and cover director at *Essence*! The ability to affirm us and create a cover concept or beauty pages based on an endless choice of Black women whose distinct beauty made them a muse for me was a cause célèbre on the truth in beauty. As much as I could envision it, I dreamt a world—casting women with gaps and gorgeous full lips and those with green eyes and cappuccino skin! From Queens with full-blown fros to those with Bantu knots or waist-length braids or rhythmic waves or bold shaved heads—imagine stepping into the studio every month with a hand-picked glam squad to work with some of the most captivating women in the world: models, actors, singers, activists, everyday gals if you will, and more. From First Lady Michelle Obama to Missy Elliott, from Naomi Campbell and Iman to Beyoncé and Angela Davis, or, or, or, check, check, check. For Yours Truly, it's always about affirming our definition of beauty and assuring us that there are none among us who will be invisible and that there can be no standard of beauty that doesn't recognize us in all of our glory. It's clear to me that all of us must guard the portals of our minds and affirm ourselves so we become our own muses and not be otherwise-minded about the beauty we possess.

AFFIRMATION

"Be ye transformed by the renewing of your mind."

—Romans 12:2

POWER POINT

"I am no longer accepting the things I cannot change. I am changing the things I cannot accept."

—Angela Davis, professor, political activist

_____ Inspirations . . .

In the Moment with Susan L. Taylor, Founder and CEO of National CARES Mentoring Movement and Editor-in-Chief Emeritus of _Essence_ Magazine, on honoring our essential needs, listening within, and choosing our best life

"We've forgotten ourselves, lost our way. Life is a gift! Self-care must become our sacrament; charity that must begin at home for us to have wellness in mind, body, and soul, to be present to God's grace and the joy of living—no matter what we face along our journey."

"For more than four decades I've been writing and speaking about the importance of discovering and honoring our essential needs. I know well how important moments of quiet are, taking time to just be still, in silence, in our anxiety-ridden world. I have learned that quiet time is the only sure pathway to balance and inner peace, wellness and joy—and that it is the most important time we must take. But still, when the stresses in my over-scheduled life press too closely around me, allowing anxiety and fear to creep in, the first things I often let go of are the very things I need most to stay strong in my faith, mind, body, and soul: morning meditation, exercise, taking five deep, slow breaths throughout, proven to relax and restore us a minute, planning healthy snacks and meals while on the run—and eating them mindfully and slowly. Living at a pace of grace is a great challenge for all of us in our technology-driven, over-connected, and frenzied world. Slowing down and taking time to restore each day what life depletes is the mighty challenge for most women. Early on, we learn that we were born to bow to the needs of others, that sacrifice and selflessness are virtues that make us worthy of love. All of us—male and female alike—are here on assignment. We were born to love, to care for "the least of these," nurture our families, advance our people, heal our world. We've forgotten ourselves, lost our way. Life is a gift! Self-care must become our sacrament; charity that must begin at home for us to have wellness in mind, body, and soul, to be present to God's grace and the joy of living—no matter what we face along our journey. Constantly attending to the unending tasks and others' needs without restoring what a culture on steroids exhausts in us is an act of self-betrayal."Disregarding our value and worth is a sure route to burnout, depression, and a host of other lifestyle illnesses. But it can also be an awakening, the slap upside our head we need to restore our self and bring our life back to balance—which is always a choice we have. It's not enough to be kind. We must learn to be kind *and* wise. Living in balance is vital to well-being, but living a balanced life doesn't just happen. We have to make an ongoing commitment to inner peace and well-being, and to living with compassion, not just for others but also for ourselves. A great gift from our Creator is our power to choose. What I appreciate most about life is that change is forever possible. As we become more vigilant guardians of our inner life, any wounds we are carrying begin to heal, and our life is transformed. We no longer allow people, institutions, or our cultural mores to speak to us so loudly we cannot hear the still, small voice of Spirit. Life is a journey, our inner walk to wholeness and fulfillment, finding our way back home to faith and the true self we've been taught to deny. Ignore your inner bidding and you risk becoming an unfulfilled impostor who gives power and governance to surrounding forces rather than the mightiest force on earth: the love of God ordering the universe, surrounding us, within us, breathing us, beating our heart. The life we are living reflects that life we have established within ourselves. Clarity and confidence emerge in the quiet. We become calm, fully present, and aware of the steps we should take, the moves we must make to live meaningful, productive, prosperous lives, which is our Creator's intention for us. We know the way to inner peace and balance. Our challenge is to close the book, leave the faith service, turn away from the screens, and practice, practice, practice living it. Begin each day giving yourself to you before giving yourself away. Make time for quiet time, for listening in. Fire the judge. Speak kindly to your precious self, as tenderly as you would to a baby. Get up and get going! Exercise. Eat (to live) a plant-based diet, and only till you are satisfied, not stuffed full. Have faith! You were born on purpose, with a purpose. Life needs you! Rebooting your life, you'll breathe new energy into your passions—focus on what you came here to give, not to get. Staying connected to the Holy Spirit strengthens and guides our lives. We smartly choose self-care and compassion for ourselves, then service to others. Our fears and insecurities evaporate. We see that we are *just right*, perfectly imperfect yet more than enough. We don't cherish the approval of others or the many beliefs and behaviors that undermine our self-discovery and wholeness. We awaken each day with gratitude filling our heart, prepared to give our best to life in appropriate measure, ever grateful for God's grace, and to our foreparents for all they withstood to make our lives of freedom and privilege possible. Growing in awareness and courage, we see who and what are destructive or nourishing to us—and we choose! And any burdens we believe we carry? We remember that we are forever in the arms of God—no matter how things may appear. With walk-on-water faith, we keep stepping, entrusting our outcomes to divine order, to the Giver of Life. Our duties and cares are handled with greater strength, clarity, and joy. Our worries are viewed as what *they* are—a call from beyond to look for the Divine Hand in all things, renew, refocus, and refine the great gift of our beautiful life."

66 I learned to focus and give my best, 100 percent excellence, to whatever I was doing at the time. Then, it did not matter what anyone else said or did not say."

—Iyanla Vanzant, author, inspirational speaker, and host of OWN TV's *Iyanla: Fix My Life*

Invest in Yourself

I don't believe in "makeovers." I don't believe the King sent any of us here "wrong." I do believe in new possibilities and self-discovery. One of my favorite examples is found in the Old Testament in the story of Queen Esther, who went through a purification process of inner and outer beauty treatments, attitudinal shifts, and was ultimately tested to prove her capability to lead and not shrink back. As we look back in the portals of history, we see that every Queen had a "temple-management team" who supported her through a process of coaching, beauty rituals, and internal work to develop and sustain the visionary leader she was destined to be. What I say to each of us is that we, too, must commit to what is essentially an investment strategy that supports us and helps us to be in full command. Everything old isn't antiquated, and the old adage "Beauty is as beauty does" still holds true, so you must not sell yourself short and fail to incorporate the people, practices, and thinking that will push, polish, and support you at your best.

As an editor, I've helped countless women explore the possibilities in beauty with the best pros in the business to show them how and where to invest in themselves, but real change always stems from within, and I can tell you, when the change is solely superficial, as in a new hairstyle, or makeup, or a change in the way one dresses, those are the women who, when you meet them later on, you see they've gone right back to the same old stuff, because they were the same person inside and didn't commit or support the change. Now I'm good, and I work with the best creative teams in the industry, but in order for the external to stick, one's internal must shift; ditto for their actions. As Queens, we should define those practices that make the most valuable deposits in our spirits and recognize that by making these investments we'll reap the benefits within and without. Assessing your beauty from this perspective will shift your self-view and cause you to consistently engage in rejuvenating practices, be it committing to monthly massages and realizing the proven benefits or enlisting the support of a life coach to give you the know-how needed to turn your desires into reality. One thing is certain: when you think about investing in yourself, don't go it alone. It's an unnecessary challenge, and it can also be difficult to hold yourself accountable. I think every gal should have support, no matter how small, to sustain her in those practices that'll keep her inner and outer beauty in the flow.

Who's on "Team You"?

When your attitude shifts, you recognize that "Her Majesty" must decide who and what will form her support. Moreover, she recognizes that it's not about what anyone else thinks of her "self-nurturing" investments but about how *she* values them. This is part of your personal agreement of unconditional love and reveals that you acknowledge your needs. It also helps you be an effective servant leader because it shows that you recognize that before you can serve others, you must take care of *home.* Today's a good day for you to turn to the "Notes to Self" pages at the end of this chapter and enter your activation steps and gauge who should be added to your temple-management team. You've already begun one with your doctor, perhaps your hairstylist, and anyone else you've enlisted to support your beauty and overall well-being. Now, why not pull out your calendar and begin to schedule time and rituals with yourself by pragmatically defining *your* private appointments? Whether it's a long milk bath or a chair massage, begin to live in support mode by anticipating your needs. I have a barre club membership and a monthly massage membership because one strengthens my focus and the other relaxes my muscles, releases tension, and opens my creative thoughts. These appointments are as essential to my internal beauty as my appointments with my hairstylist, my dental hygienist, and anyone else on my temple-management team. There's no better time to invest in your life and move assertively into the care practices you desire. Start by throwing away your wish list; begin the checklist and, when and where applicable, put a date on it. Don't look in the rearview mirror, you'll crash your determination, and please refuse the thinking that says, "I don't have time," "I can't." It's the most direct route to stagnation. Take the road untraveled to your best life, explore the possibilities, get to know yourself, be inspired, and activate the plan to invest in you.

When you're clear, you don't wait for opportunity to find you—you create it!

Mikki-ism

Being intentional in your life really comes down to possessing an instinct to thrive and being deeply engaged in your well-being. Don't wait for another 365 to turn around the sun, otherwise known as your birthday, to celebrate the truth of who you are. It's more than chronological; it's constitutional! If you need some Webster for it, here goes: "The fundamental makeup of something, inherent in, authorized"— own it and recognize that you are to be so intentional concerning you. Feeling great and looking great go hand in hand. In the meantime, honor the Queen in you. For example, if you like the way your temple feels when you get up from a massage table, don't wait for another gift certificate; sign up for a plan. Queens don't belong on "well-being welfare." Answer the call: you make sure everyone else is accommodated in the kingdom—don't neglect the Queen! If your body needs to answer the lure of a nap on Saturday when everyone else is running a marathon to-do list, step to it. Why not even dress for the journey? Slip into a fabulous caftan and have your pillow drift. The reality of it is this: You may have nothing to do with what's going on around you, but you have everything to do with what's going on inside of you. And if your cup is empty, you just ought to know you cannot give what you don't have.

So get your zzz's! Investing in restorative time for self is not an option; it is nonnegotiable! And in this insta-age where everyone is in a hurry, don't be guilty. You don't want an insta-life—it's meaningless, elusive. Insta-experiences are gone in a heartbeat. It's like the difference between sex and making love; one is done before you know it, and the other is worth the journey! The real gratification that comes from investing in yourself is always worth the time.

It's also worth noting that the Word instructs us to "lay aside every weight that easily besets you"—in other words, get rid of those things that easily hold you back and, where necessary, unlearn those attitudes that hinder the Queen in you and complicate your life. As Vanzant puts it, "Clean up your energy!" A lot of us struggle with prioritizing our energies, taxing ourselves beyond measure by saying "yes" to everything within our power. I've been guilty of this, too, and I had to learn the hard way that this kind of behavior is unrealistic, often crippling, and that I cannot deliver excellence from a place of *lack*. So I had to honestly face my limits and stop accepting twenty tasks when I know I'm only able to do ten *well*. I had to learn the courage to lovingly say "no" with complete confidence to those things that would pull me off track so I could say "yes" to that which would keep me on purpose and, by doing so, stake a deeper claim in my own life. Whatever your personal challenge is, acknowledge it and address it so you can attend to those practices that enhance your well-being.

Establish Your Celebration Circle

The King desires that you be surrounded, supported, and celebrated in the journey, and he has packaged this in the Word by instructing us to "exhort and encourage one another, rejoice when they rejoice, weep when they weep." Again, you can't take this journey alone and unsupported, so don't move through life as a Queen in isolation. Research has proven that deprivation of empowering relationships results in detrimental behavior, limited thinking, and daunted growth. Increasingly in this high-tech, low-touch age, this form of loneliness or lack of community is becoming a modern-day health challenge with indications that it's a predictor of poor health. It's also the primary problem of 80 percent of those seeking psychiatric support. The abundant life will elude you if you don't enlist divine thinking and the proper support to see you through. I know you need a support circle, for even Jesus chose twelve, a president has a cabinet, a chairwoman has a team. When it comes to life, you need a celebration circle, and if you haven't established who's on it, be about the business of ensuring or identifying those who support you through thick and thin because supportive relationships promote your growth, shore up your inner beauty, and keep you on purpose. In selecting this critical circle of celebrants, be choosy—everybody can't hang. Don't hallucinate in your choices and imagine the dolls and the guys are someone that they're not. Don't make excuses for those who exhibit bad behavior in your life; that's not wise. Know enough not to put your joy up for sale! "Your hopes, dreams, fears, and desires are not safe with every single person that you have a great time with," says Lauren Lake, family lawyer and host of *Lauren Lake's Paternity Court*. So it's not about inviting incapable people into your core circle. Life is challenging enough as it is, and you need a team of "rough riders," a.k.a. celebrants who are test-worthy and there for you no matter what the season is in your life, who'll not only help you celebrate your successes but also help you to shine even in the dark hour of challenge, who'll counsel you with wisdom, tell you when you're going in the wrong direction, Samaritan you when you've been knocked down, and stand with you against all odds on the road to your comeback. This is how the Queen wears the crown. She understands that in her court, there's a support system of like-minded advocates and accountability partners, and together they love and rejoice over one another no matter what life shows them.

Food for Thought

There are things that money can't buy and that possessions can't satisfy, but a good friend is invaluable. I'm blessed to have those in my life that I can call "friend," and I don't take it lightly. We love each other no matter what. We disagree, get crunchy, and stand firm for what we believe in, tell each other the truth when we like it and when we don't, but we've got each other's back, always and forever. I believe the best relationships are those that are cultivated over time. In a sense, they're like courtships, full of shared experiences that allow you to know and love one another. Thirty-five years ago, I married one such friend, and I don't ever want to know life without him. My sister, Candace, though the youngest, is really both big sister and my ride-or-die-for-life friend, and her love and sage spiritual and practical advice is my wealth. My brother, Michael, is my "greatness guide," and I love him for pushing me beyond my comfort zone, shutting down my pity parties, and cheering me from level to level and so much more. My dearest friend Pamela rescued me in a store where she was the manager as I was trying to make a return over fifteen years ago, and she and I are so tight you'd think we were born twins. In fact, one day when she joked that she was going to quit me, I said no, she wasn't; if one of us showed up before God, He'd ask, "Where's the other one?" And Ms. Sandra Martin, we've been together close to forty years, and actress Marlene Dietrich could have been speaking of her when she said, "A good friend is someone you can call at four a.m." I know she's there for me, and the same holds true in return. There are others I could describe who form my celebration circle, but the bottom line is this: if you've got a core circle, cherish them; if you don't, make room.

About Us

As I travel the country, I'm hearing more and more that we are having great difficulty befriending one another as women, and this should not be so. If the ancestors could be brought here from different villages, speaking different languages, and form communities and families and give birth to generations of powerful women through the ages who supported one another, we have got to do better. We should be growing together in love, both through triumph and in struggle. I think one of the many reasons we have trouble creating and sustaining strong female relationships is that we've been misinformed about what true friendship is, and as a result, we don't choose wisely. We also forget that everyone is not destined to be a friend. Some are simply associates, and when we confuse their identity or role in our lives, we get into trouble. Every gal should have a set of requirements for friendship just like anything else that holds value in her life.

Here's a basic friend ID:

- Trustworthy

- Honest

- Consistent

- Dependable

- Supportive

- Inspiring

- Loves unconditionally

you have to develop is the honesty to ask yourself: Am I the kind of friend I'd want for someone else? Am I there only when it's convenient for me? How consistent am I? Am I the person I'd want as a friend during the tough times?" Dr. Sherry says. Clearly there's a need for us to check ourselves as the best relationships are reciprocal. This is where character is put to the test. "You have to possess the courage to be the friend you need and not fall prey to the mediocrity that exists," Lake points out. Experts like Dr. Sherry and others also believe that a lot of time we get in our own way because we're not only afraid of getting to know people; we're also afraid of people getting to know us—"because there's a fear of rejection and issues that may emerge, so we wear the mask, too," she concludes. Again, herein lies another opportunity to know your value and not audition for the approval of others. Moreover, it should encourage you to hold yourself accountable for all the qualities you desire in others.

> 66 Some people are keepers, some are just drive-by friends, but a real friend will stand the test of time."
>
> —Dr. Sherry Blake, clinical psychologist

The Last Word

Everybody does not earn the right to be on your inner circle. "You want people to be a part of your circle who'll challenge your thinking and push you and be happy for you," says Dr. Sherry. They have to be women who'll provide unconditional love regardless of your circumstances, who'll pour wisdom into your life while valuing that which you pour in return.

According to Lauren, every gal needs a mother or mother figure, "someone that has your best interest at heart even when you don't," and "we all need that sister friend, that we feel can be the confidant, so much so that you can give her the keys to the vault." Without question, each of us needs a friend who's spiritually and physically health conscious to keep us grounded in our faith and on our toes. Requirements vary, and they are different for each of us at various times in our lives, but the bottom line is this: it's not the number of friends; it's the quality of those friends you have. Finally, know that your friendship circle is a lifeline, "a living, breathing call to action," as Lake says. Make it count!

POWER POINT

God doesn't have to prepare the blessing. He has to prepare you for the blessing!

Commune with the King

Support comes in many forms, but to me there's nothing like that which comes from prayer. I love a good, spirit-nourishing conversation, and it's a great joy to be able to get on the royal hotline! I also find that given the hectic pace and, at times, the assaults of daily life at capacity that I need the restorative communication that comes from consulting with the King, so I boldly go to the throne of grace for my get-together on the regular. In fact, kicking off my day in prayer changes the tempo of everything, and closing each day out in thanksgiving keeps me reminded that God is on my side. Moreover, consulting Him in prayer throughout the day is what orders life. This is the all-access status that means everything. I've called on Him on my knees as well as flat on my back from an ambulance after falling headlong down a flight of stairs and fracturing several ribs; I've talked to him in the church as well as onstage, and I hesitated not to give thanks prior to entering the operating room for removal of an adrenal tumor. I remember the staff saying they'd never seen anyone come into that room smiling, but I was joyful as I knew the King had me covered. After being diagnosed with an adrenal tumor the size of a newborn's head, I began an affirmation journal so I would stay in agreement with Him concerning my well-being and not allow my mind to entertain fearful thoughts that my body would carry out! I continued to work; at that time I was scriptwriting the annual Essence Black Women in Hollywood Awards. By faith I had successful laparoscopic surgery, which removed an eight-centimeter tumor, despite the fact that the cutoff size for this type of surgery is six centimeters. This is the power of prayer without doubt.

I spend time in the presence of the King for the kind of strength and direction I need to be my highest self and to execute leadership over the things I've been divinely assigned to do. I know that He wants the best for me and has plans to prosper me mentally, spiritually, and physically, and all I have to do is seek his wisdom, especially when adversity stops by to threaten the truth. For me, prayer has been the place where my best battles have been fought and won! Though Queen Esther was purified and nurtured for twelve months, nothing refined her inner beauty like adversity. How you handle adversity can impact your beauty for keeps—from stress lines and hair loss to crippling low self-esteem—if you *let* it. Again, perspective has a lot to do with it, and I've found that it is in adversarial times that we experience growth the most, and I'm learning, like King David, to not only face the giants of adversity but to run out and meet them with divine direction. I'm getting strengthened by my conversations with the King to not let fear get in the way because the equalizing thing about fear is this: if you don't put it away, it has the potential to put you away! I've long been clear that I have a choice—to either trust God without measure or resort to my own limited knowledge—and I'm bent on choosing the former and tapping into the kind of life force information that's key to being at my best. When you think about it, there are all kinds of prayers. The main thing is to engage in them.

In the Moment with Ledisi, Singer, Songwriter, Actress, on celebrating her beauty and self-growth and honoring her soul's purpose

"You can not like me and what I choose to do; you don't have to like my music, you don't have to like my hair, but you do have to respect me."

"I'm another option of *beauty*, I'm another version for you. I don't compare myself to other women, I don't compete in that way, I just be Ledisi. I don't look for validation from others, I look for it from myself. I'll never be like Mary J., I'll never be like Solange or Beyoncé, I'm not trying to be them. I want to be my version of sexy and beautiful and hot and chocolate and earthy and jazzy and funky. I want to be all those things as I like to change it up. In fact, I had to create options for myself, because no one was giving that to me, but that internal pull was saying, 'I want that and I'm going to have it.' Now everyone has more options because of me standing up for me. I'm going to own that! Sometimes we just need to be still because the world is pulling on us and it's even harder now. We have all these avenues to give and we don't give back to ourselves. We give it to everybody else and there's nothing to pull from. Then you're exhausted and you don't know why, and you're eating and you don't know why, you don't want to work out and you don't know why, and you want to sleep and you don't know why. I love getting older and I think learning to say 'no' helped me know the significance of understanding my value. As a young person, you don't get that right away. It comes by being observant and being still and listening more. Stillness is hard for me, but it's important as it helps me to be aware. What I say to us: demand time to be with yourself. I say 'demand' because it's hard to make these moments, so you have to be adamant about knowing, 'I need this time for me, I need time to explore, time even to just look in the mirror.' Even if you just get off of social media, clean out your closet, read a book, take time to explore for yourself knowledge or spirituality, not just getting your nails done. It's so hard being women, and then being a Black woman is harder because we're being judged constantly, we're competing constantly, we wear so many hats, but we never ever say,

'I'm going to demand this moment for me.' I call that a check-in when you demand moments for yourself. 'Ledisi' is a Nigerian Yoruba word that means 'to bring forth,' and I bring forth excellence. When you hear my name, you know it will be a moment, it will be excellence, as that is my primary goal. Everything I do must be done well, it must look well, it must feel well. I'm becoming a better actress and a better writer. I already know I can sing, I already know I can perform—thank you God for that—and I do it well because You want it to be done well, but I want to learn. Learning is what makes me a better performer and better at anything I touch: a better giver, a better woman, a better overall human being to add onto this world. I have learned when you give back without expectation it comes back to you, and helping people has been the best reward of my life. Then there's the unspoken thing: prayer is everything. I couldn't sing like I do, write like I do, act like I do, give like I do—I couldn't do anything that I do if I didn't have that spiritual strength that comes with knowing God and having my own personal relationship."

POWER POINT

Charity? Make sure it starts with you. More than any verbal declaration of self-love, the careful choices you make regarding your temple truly affirm how you feel about yourself.

Rituals for a Modern-Day Queen

Every Queen should incorporate those practices that nurture her beauty and well-being. Restorative practices are essential for the busy life you lead as they polish and replenish you while giving you some essential time for self. More than pampering functions, they also open up a pathway to hear within, draw close to your desires, and envision bringing them to life. Don't miss the opportunity to nurture your body, mind, and spirit by failing to commit to the rituals that affirm you. Getting started is so simple—all you need is a few ideas (which you'll add to of course!) and the determination to carry them out. Trust me, they matter. Here are some ways to make the connection:

Sybaritic Bliss

There's nothing like the experience of a healing bath. I love those where I really get to close the door and honor the Queen in me. Oprah once told me that bubble baths are part of her ritual to get centered before going to work. For me it's the way to close down the day or kick-start a "Self-Seduction Saturday," SSS. (Shortly after writing my first book, *Self-Seduction: Your Ultimate Path to Inner and Outer Beauty*, I determined every Saturday would be my day to self-nurture.) It's also the place where I meditate and where great ideas spring forth just through this self-nurturing practice of getting still. I know it's important that I make time to pour into myself after giving me away all week, so I'm asking you to prioritize yourself with this ritual, even if only once a week, and stay committed. To this day, I keep finding new ways to take bathing to the next level depending on my needs and desires. To relax and reduce inflammation, I add essential oils of lavender, ylang-ylang, safflower oil (which contains linoleic acid to reduce inflammation), and Epsom salts to my bath. If I want to escape, oceanic-inspired soaks like Crabtree & Evelyn's La Source Revitalising Mineral Muscle Soak take me away. To nourish and soothe, in goes a cup of milk and a few drops of sage or sandalwood oil; to detox, seaweed, which contains minerals that increase circulation and move toxins out of the lymphatic system. When I want to luxuriate and hydrate, in goes Jo Malone's Red Roses Bath Oil. No matter the ingredients, I always incorporate some extras to engage my mind, body, and spirit:

- Bath pillow
- Bath tray
- Jazz
- Candle

- A good read
- Heated towel rack

Time Out

Who doesn't like a goodie bag at the end of a great gathering? Next time you have the girlfriends over, why not make it extra special by giving them a little gift of "peace and solitude" to help them begin their own sybaritic ritual? "Bath-Time Bliss Bags" are the perfect way to do so and are ideal treats to give busy women like yourself. Here's how: hit a craft shop for small cellophane bags and ribbon, buy scented bath salts by the ounce at Lush stores or Whole Foods (lavender is a great choice), and fill each one with six to eight ounces and a special message, and you will have given the best gift of all, time for self. How thoughtful are you!

Pleasure Principles

Each of us has meaningful ways in which we honor the pleasures of a good Saturday. I look forward to those Saturdays when I have nothing on the calendar to attend to and can spend some time helping myself to the pleasures of the day, from self-nurturing to enjoying time with my loves. With no wake-up call, no alarm, and the pleasure of just waking up when my body is ready to start the day, I ease in. As I do each and every morning, I greet the day in meditation and prayer; it's my way of mind-keeping and tending my mental and spiritual fitness. I love snuggling in with hubby, giggling like children over times past and present, the young'uns, and more. Saturday is also the day I look to do my beauty maintenance: clean the makeup brushes, maybe do a light scrub, get a massage and/or pedicure, and have a slow bath. This is also my time to do a good wardrobe check: dry cleaning, shoe repairs, and a visit to the tailor for any alteration needs. Sometimes I just engage in what the experts call a "moving meditation" (I call it "puttering"), and it's good to my spirit to just move around doing this and that as I please. However you like to spend Saturday, make it count and indulge yourself in pleasures great and small because this is your life and you owe it to yourself to make sure it's centered on what brings you joy.

Pillow Talk

I think sleep is the most awesome beauty treatment in the world, and I've tried enough treatments to know! When we skimp on sleep, we're really cheating on ourselves and cutting short a divine-inspired period of rest and healing—just check out Psalm 23:2. The King is concerned about your rest and has created your body to heal itself during sleep. No wonder it's called "beauty sleep." When we come up short, we see the telltale signs through compromised energy, dark circles, and irritability. We also miss the big picture taking place behind the scenes, which adds up to a weakened immune system and, over time, poor muscle tone and belly fat (due to the stress hormone known as cortisol). If stepping away from the world and hitting the pillow is a challenging ritual, rethink its value to your course and get comfortable calling it a day. Think of it like you would a trip to a destination spa: it's a journey, one that you've paid for, looked forward to, and are prepared to enjoy for all it's worth.

Be intentional:

- Don't drink caffeinated beverages late in the day as that will surely create a busy mind and keep you from shutting it down.
- Establish a sleep-inducing ritual, such as taking an aromatherapy bath (incorporating essential oils that calm and relax, e.g., chamomile).
- Invest in a good mattress, one that supports your body and enhances your sleep.
- Don't watch television or work in bed—that's contrary to your intention.
- Don't carry your enemies, bills, or disappointments, etc., to bed with you—that's the antithesis of a mind at rest!
- Seduce your mind with a playlist of environmental sounds to drift by.

Remember sleep is meant to be a restorative experience, so don't undermine it. Genius and rest go together best!

Starry Nights

Experts say we spend one-third of our lives sleeping. Therefore your bedroom should be a complete sanctuary where you decompress, dream, love, and rejuvenate the Queen that you are. Why not:

- Establish a signature scent to enhance your serenity?
- Incorporate dimmers or antique lamps with sensuous lighting?
- Add a chaise lounge or settee?
- Make your bed a vessel, with the most inviting linens and luxurious pillows?

Sounds divine no?

Hands On

"Beauty is as beauty does," as the saying goes. Well, I think one of the most luxurious beauty dos you should make is to incorporate a self-massage into your daily ritual. Keeping it real, you do have to apply something lovely post bath or shower, so why not make it count? This is when more is more. Why not kick your day off or close it out using an amazing massage oil to enhance your well-being? You're certainly worth it. For example, why not blend your own? All you need is a good base oil like almond, jojoba, or sesame oil, and then it's simply about adding the essential oil(s) of your choosing based on your kneads and desires. Here's what can be found on my oil bar:

- **Neroli:** Calming.
- **Rose:** Comforting, stress-relieving.
- **Grapefruit:** Rejuvenating; counters jet lag.
- **Cypress:** Sharpens mental focus, relieves fatigue.
- **Combo fave, rosemary and grapefruit:** Energy-boosting.

Note: Essential oils should never be applied directly to your skin as they can cause irritation. When creating a massage oil, add ten to twelve drops of the essential oil to an ounce of base oil. Voilà.

Transporting Pleasures

Don't think you have to get on a plane to be transported and, equally important, don't negate the value of small rituals that enhance your journey. I've
spent an afternoon in Brazil via Pandora's best bossa nova music, enjoyed
the scented wonders of the Caribbean with my Diptyque Jasmin candle, and
sailed off the coast of Montauk under the influence of a sea-inspired bath gel
like that of Lancôme's Savon Fraîchelle—all within my domain. Experts refer
to simple pleasures like these as "sensory integration" (the ability to take in
information through your senses—touch, movement, smell, vision, hearing—
and make a meaningful response). Sensory integration also helps to expand
your vision space while reminding you of the deeper value of seemingly light-
hearted experiences that bring you joy. What's required? A mind-set that's
ready to escape, no packing necessary!

Turn Up the Heat

At the end of a long day in heels, nothing's sweeter than a foot soak—unless,
of course, it's a foot soak accompanied by a self-heating foot scrub. I love a
little mindlessness before I tuck in, especially on those days when everyone,
including my feet, has been clamoring for attention. What feels therapeutic
and luxurious is closing that bathroom door with a "do not disturb" mind-set
and massaging in a heated scrub like Bliss Hot Salt Scrub to warm, exfoliate,
and invigorate my senses with its oils of eucalyptus and rosemary. After a
good soak, I'm ready to call it day, with baby-soft feet as a bonus through this
ritual that tends to my "kneads."

Multi-Masking

A weekly purifying clay mask or a hydrating sheet mask at the end of the day
is a restorative ritual with skin-renewing results. It's also a relaxing way to get
still. You can create your own mask at home from such natural ingredients
as honey, yogurt, egg whites, and oatmeal, and target areas of your face by
adding specific ingredients to treat your different needs, e.g., to check oil,
hydrate, tighten, etc. You can also add essential oils like mint to infuse your

senses. Beauty gal that I am, I also like checking out masks from beauty hot spots, dermatological skin care lines, and destination spas. Several years ago, I visited the Blue Lagoon spa in Reykjavík, Iceland, and among the many therapeutic treatments I experienced was their world-renowned facial composed of the region's deep-cleansing white mud and glow-boosting, patented algae. Today these iconic picks, the Silica Mud Mask and Algae Mask, can be purchased online at www.shop-usa.bluelagoon.com. I'm also a fan of rejuvenating sheet masks like SK-II Facial Treatment Masks, which hydrate and immediately improve my skin texture, giving it that much-preferred "vacation glow." The key to masking, as with any other beauty ritual, is to (A) renew and restore and (B) spend time with yourself.

Soft Serve

I'm all for a good detox plan, but also find beneficial the ritual of detoxing my skin by dry-brushing with a natural-bristle body brush weekly before showering. Starting at my feet, I swiftly brush upwards in the direction of my heart in long sweeping strokes. Dry-brushing, which removes dead skin cells, leaving your body ultrasmooth and glowing, also has the following benefits:

- Boosts circulation
- Boosts lymphatic drainage and excretion of wastes
- Invigorating/energizing

So do your body and your internal beauty a favor by picking up a long-handle body brush and making this easy detox a part of a morning ritual.

Refresh Your Soul

Getting still through meditation is essential for balancing your spiritual and emotional resiliency. Through travel, I've experienced my share of great destinations for this purposeful ritual, from the sacred Indian grounds near White Sands, New Mexico, where it's so quiet you can hear the power lines overhead, to the stillness of a French castle high upon a hill in the South of France. But whether I'm destination bound or not, I make it a point to meditate *every* morning. Taking this time to get still and meditate before daybreak allows me to visualize my intentions, prioritize, purge any thoughts that are getting in my way, own what's real and release what's not, and remind myself of my truth. Every gal should make time for this ritual as it has residual benefits that you can bank on!

Rock Steady

Research has proven that rocking is therapeutic as it taps into a pleasure center in the brain. It's a favored ritual of Queens in the know and is becoming increasingly popular in mind-body work to calm the nervous system, relax muscles, and bring your body into balance. You can invoke this healing motion anywhere and at any pace to soothe your spirit.

POWER POINT
Take five. In the midst of serving everyone else in your life, be sure to place your name on the list.

66 The ultimate measure of a woman is not where she stands in moments of comfort and convenience, but where she stands at times of challenge and controversy."

—Dr. Martin Luther King Jr., minister, activist, humanitarian, legend

Are you standing on the promises of God or standing by, waiting to see what's going to happen? Don't be on standby—show up ready!

Mikki-ism

In the Moment with Lisa Nichols, Motivational Speaker, Author, CEO of Motivating the Masses, on self-esteem, personal care, and standing strong

"There's no lifeline that God didn't already give me. I wake up enough—smart enough, young enough, brilliant enough—and before I check anything on social media, I first need to like myself."

"I decided years ago to stop putting my self-esteem on the judgment table when something occurs. My esteem is not available to my circumstances, to who's in office, my love-life situation, my bank account, what the scale says when I climb up on it—it's *not* available! It didn't happen in one aha moment, it happened in layers of awareness. It started with me measuring myself against other people and then realizing that comparison was the thief of all joy. Every time I compared myself to someone else, I came up short, until I realized that there is no comparison to the unique value that I bring. I learned that my self-esteem was given to me at birth. I was born jubilant, I was born joyful, I was born curious, I was born adventurous, I was born with strong characteristics, like a fully loaded car. Externally, I came through school with mocha skin, full lips, round hips, kinky hair. I wasn't a beauty queen. And those very same things to this day are things I love most about me, and I wouldn't trade it for the world, but I had to learn how to dance with it. I've been very intentional about who God designed me to be and very mindful of not getting in the way of that. I know that self-care is not selfish, self-care is your responsibility to your future. I'm adamant about this because this one took me the longest to learn and it's the lesson that has almost killed me several times. It's arrogant to believe that the world around us cannot survive without us! I'm a single mom and a CEO and I travel over two hundred days a year, and so self-care is the thing that I thought last about. Then I realized there's a divine unique calling on your life that only you can fulfill. Your responsibility to that divine calling is to be in self-care enough so you can be awake, aware, and energized enough to fulfill it. Self-care is also a responsibility to not serve people from your cup but from your saucer, your overflow. I've known great opposition and adversity, and while in it I still had to show up and inspire the world! But challenge doesn't define my character, it uncovers parts of my character that I didn't know I had. It's my challenges that have confirmed the woman I get to become. Tethered to that is my unwavering, nonnegotiable, unquestionable faith. There've been times when I've not been on my knees, I've been on my face crying out to God and saying, 'I know what you are to me and it hurts to be in this space, but I know the light at the end of the tunnel is not a train.' When you know you already got the victory, you just got to walk the walk, so I nourish my body, take my B12, and do what I have to do so I can get the walk. What's critical to owning my life is knowing there's no lifeline that God didn't already give me. I wake up *enough*—smart enough, young enough, brilliant enough—and before I check anything on social media, I first need to *like* myself. What's also critical is to set an intention to live a life that creates few to no regrets when you're ready to sit down. To know the distinction of when you're asking for permission to be you and when you're giving the world notice that this is how bright my light is. Lastly, to recognize that when it comes to your life accomplishment, your life declaration, that there's a responsibility on your breath to inspire those around you to be better. That must call you out of your fear because that honor calling says that you've been selected to show up and give the world this contribution. I made a list of ten declarations of who I choose to be and I laminated them and put them in my shower because I needed to know when I'm butt naked who I am declaring to be!"

Build Your Spiritual Muscle

When I first started kickboxing, I couldn't keep my balance, let alone put up a good fight, but I was determined to not let it get the best of me and to become *great*—not good, but great at it. One of the most valuable lessons my trainer taught me was that it wasn't just about showing up for my sessions with the hopes of getting better, but putting in the necessary time on the sidelines to strengthen my muscles and improve my core. I'll never forget what is, in a sense, a true-life application for empowered women. No one is exempt from challenge, but that which tests us not only shows what we're made of but also offers us an opportunity to grow and become stronger at our core. I've been through enough to tell you the truth and I know for certain it's in the face of challenge that we have the capacity to grow the most, and you don't want to just "go through"; you want to "*grow* through." I've learned that challenges and adversity are where preparation meets opportunity. In order to show up ready, we must lift the weights of life to build the kind of strength that goes the distance. The spiritual strength I possess today has made me the woman that I am, and I wouldn't take anything for the capabilities that I now possess as they have been hard won through patience, prayer, endurance, and graciousness. Dealing with narcissistic people in the work of empowering Black women was at times devaluing and tormenting, but it compelled me to keep going and move "self" out of the way because it wasn't about me; it was about *us*, and so purpose took precedence over pressure, personalities, and pettiness. There's an old saying that speaks to purpose: "Gold is put in the furnace so it can be purified." Every hurdle that you leap, you land a stronger woman on the other side. You never know what's ahead of you or what you're being prepared for, but you want to show up ready. When I think back on the things I tripped over, I know they were light stuff compared to what lay in my future. I also know that you cannot lead without knowing humility. Humility is a virtue, and long before I had the title I developed the character to serve. Home is where you learn who you are and begin to develop the kind of character traits that will serve you well. If I had not learned selflessness, kindness, courtesy, and the compassion to recognize that hurt people hurt others, I would never have succeeded or had the capacity to deal with challenge and adversity, nor would I have learned to love others from my heart and not from my hurt. My mother used to tell me as I was coming of age, "Don't cut your nose off to spite your face." Whew, that was always a heavy dose of wisdom for me, and I can tell you that I cringed whenever she said this because it meant that I was about to make a hasty, perhaps spiteful decision, where the results would cost me more than I was prepared to pay. Eventually I got the lesson and began to "grow up gracefully." Nowadays we often talk about aging gracefully, but very rarely do you hear anyone talk about "growing gracefully." Growing gracefully means mastering the art of being humble and patient. The New Testament gives us many a master class on both and how they are fundamental to living our best lives. In fact, one of my favorite passages says, "Let patience have her perfect work." In other words, don't do anything to hinder or limit your patience, and by doing this, you'll grow, perfect your attitude, and increase your wisdom. By practicing this, I've learned the value of not reacting to short-term circumstances with long-term measures. In terms of being humble, it's part of the check-and-balance system that keeps me anchored and focused. I'm about service, not status. I recognize that my every ability is divinely given unto a purpose, so far be it from me to become puffed-up or reactionary about anything I've been assigned to do. What I learned is if you serve with excellence, you'll make a name for yourself.

POWER POINT

When you put your faith in the right place, you don't have to worry about the future.

In the early days at *Essence*, we did it all. I remember our weekly meetings with Susan L. Taylor when she was fashion and beauty editor where we developed stories on legal pads and went out to execute them on photo shoots as a small but visionary team that was composed of Sandra Martin, Ionia Dunn Lee, Yours Truly, and Sister Susan. Nobody talked about what was or wasn't on her job description; we worked under the edict of "we put this magazine out for and about ourselves," and what drove us was passion and purpose! Not to negate one's value, but what helped me to stay humble to this day is determining that purpose is of more importance than my ego. I can remember being on a cover shoot with Aretha Franklin and actor Glynn Turman and having to run across the Pacific Coast Highway to get ribs for the Queen of Soul to save the shot before the sun went down. Ego would have said no, but purpose said yes! I tied Diana Ross's shoes on a shoot long before Suzanne de Passe hired me to freelance for her as a stylist, watched Iman's daughter Zulekha while she was in makeup, and went the extra mile through many a publicist's giant ego to get to their talent, who, mind you, were not egotistical, not thinking I was too good for any of it. Didn't matter that it wasn't in my job description—it was in my character to serve. Funny how it all worked out. Years later, I was asked to write my own job description!

Staying humble takes more than mere human effort. It comes from living by faith. Challenges, no matter what form they take, personal or professional, give you experience, develop your patience, increase your wisdom, and build your spiritual muscle. They help you to learn over time how to master yourself, trust God, and execute sound judgment.

"Do unto others as you would have them do unto you."

—Matthew 7:12

POWER POINT

None of us are strangers to adversity, but if you let it take you prisoner, it will hold you captive. Don't give in, give up, or give out.

So, sis, take the challenge master class whenever it's in session so you can move beyond your comfort zone and grow deeper into your power zone. You don't want to sit on the throne and not know how to own it! Nor do you want to be caught in a challenge trying to "get ahold of yourself." You want to be the one who knows how to hold it down and remain steady, so you must develop the necessary strength and calm ahead of time.

"Broken moments can be your reality, but they are not your truth."

—Sheri Riley, author, life strategist

Stop walking by sight and walk by faith. If it were that visible, everybody would get it!

Mikki-ism

POWER POINT

Don't be more afraid of challenge, risk, and opposition than you are of fulfilling your dreams.

BANNER DAY RX

Make it a practice to note one thing you're grateful for each day and place it in the "notes" section on your phone. Refer to it during those times when you're waiting in line at the bank or the market. "Take five" with it when you're pressed for patience; by all means reflect on it and know that you are blessed.

Don't maintain. MAXIMIZE!

Mikki-ism

_____ Inspirations . . .

In the Moment with Sheryl Lee Ralph, Actress, Singer, and Activist, on self-awareness, the importance of being kind, and daring to be fearless!

"I'm able to stay centered, validated, and refrain from auditioning for the approval of others because I approve of myself, doggone it! I'm not waiting for you to tell me I'm okay, I know I'm okay!"

"My parents were always, always reminding me of how valuable I was and that I was important and had something to offer. I never quite knew what that was as a child, but I do know I felt it. What I love most about my beauty is the fact that I didn't give up on it! When I was little, my nickname was Ugmo! I was the original 'but her face'—'Oh, great girl, but her face!' My nose was too big, my lips were too thick, I was darker than the paper bag, so there were all these things they were trying to tell you that said you were ugly, but my mother would tell me I was beautiful and I believed her. And without the help of a knife or a scalpel or anything I have become the woman people see now. So what if I'm not the one you chose, too bad for you. You will realize and you will come back, and oftentimes they do come right back! I'm able to stay centered, validated, and refrain from auditioning for the approval of others because I approve of myself, doggone it! I'm not waiting for you to tell me I'm okay, I know I'm okay! People spend too much time being unkind. I had a mentor in actress Virginia Capers, who said to me once, 'Be as nice as you can, be as kind as you can to as many people as you can, because the same a** you kick today, you may have to kiss tomorrow.' She was so good to me from the moment I met her as one of the top ten college women in America. She stuck with me till the day she died. I remember one time things were going so good for me when I was in *Dreamgirls* and she said to me, 'There's this thing called ego, never let it get the best of you, because all ego wants to do is trip you, so do not give in to ego.' There have been moments in this industry where I have simply dared to tell the truth. When I won the Independent Spirit Award, I said, 'Yes, I am Black, I am female, I am talented, and I could do so much more if you all just gave me the chance, if you all just wrote the role for me, what couldn't I do?' I'll never ever forget what my grandmother used to say to me: 'Sheryl Lee Ralph, when you enter the room, the whole race comes with you. So, if you go out there looking awful, you just bought awfulness with you, but if you go out there bringing your best, trying to always present your best, then you brought the best of us with you.' It's my truth."

66 **Y**ou have to determine what is valuable and what is not so you know how to build and carry forward."

—Dorothy Height, educator, civil and women's rights activist

_____ Inspirations . . .

In the Moment with Yolanda Adams, Grammy Award–winning gospel singer, producer, and entrepreneur, on gratitude, spiritual strength, and self-discovery

"I don't like the word 'reinvention' because it means that you have to start all over and God made you authentic and original, and why would you want to reinvent something He already perfected?"

"I start off my day with a grateful heart, through meditation and prayer. Gratitude is so important, and when you realize you have a whole lot of things to be thankful for—I'm walking, I'm talking, nobody has to push me around, nobody has to feed me through a tube—you realize, 'I have it pretty good.' I have learned to build my spiritual muscle not just on prayers and thanksgiving but in my daily activities. Spirituality is not how calm your day is or calm your life is; spirituality is how you manage your life in the tough times. Can you be grateful when everything around you looks impossible? If all your bills are paid, you have no debt, all your friends are loving you, and everything is good, the grateful part of you comes through; you don't need faith for that. You need faith for the impossible. By faith I can say this, too, shall pass, and as this passes, I will learn from this and I will grow from this and I'm going to be the best me that I can possibly be as a result of this. If I concentrate on the joy of the journey as opposed to what I think the journey is taking me to, I understand the providence of an all-seeing, all-knowing God because everything I'm doing and moving toward doing, He's already set a plan for. I'm not going to second-guess his plan, I'm not going to overstep the plan, I'm going to walk in the plan because as I walk in the plan I not only find out about things

He put in me—how wise I am, how equipped I am—I find out things about Him and that there's nothing that He hasn't already equipped me for, so why you tripping, Yolanda? There's a *discovery* that happens every day of your life. I don't like the word 'reinvention' because it means that you have to start all over and God made you authentic and original, and why would you want to reinvent something He already perfected? At age fifty-five, I understand I'm given more territory, that my tent and my borders are bigger and wider and broader and more global now. My favorite scripture is Amos 9:13, from the *Message* translation, and it talks about how things in your life are going to happen so fast your head will swim, and it's going to be one thing after another, blessings upon blessings, and whenever I think we've achieved this and there's no more, I go back to that scripture because there's always more. There's always more to do, more to give, more to see, more to learn. When I deal with challenges and situations that look like setbacks and failures, I get in the Word and look at scriptures that are totally against what it looks like. I know God is too big for this to be the end of it. He's too big for that to be my legacy. The Word says God gives you life and He will give you abundance till it overflows. I know that if I'm not at the point of the promise, something else is about to break forth!"

AFFIRMATION

" 'For I know the plans I have for you,' declares the Lord, 'plans
to prosper you . . . plans to give you hope and a future.' "
—Jeremiah 29:11

66 God has given you something that takes you out of your comfort zone, and the way to discover it is to get in it and ride the wave of life."

—Lauren Lake

Dream and Discover

What sends you over the moon or makes your heart skip a beat? Don't think for minute that this kind of fulfillment isn't important to your inner and outer beauty! Whatever stimulates you and pushes you to be at your best must be realized. But what is it that makes us hold back on our dreams? Fear! According to Sonia Jackson Myles, founder and CEO of The Sister Accord, LLC, so much of the fear we experience is deposited in us by our parents, and we have generational cycles of baggage that keep being passed on, and they have to be erased so we have the courage to go on. "The fears our parents have or what we're told we can't do from a young age prevents us from believing we deserve to dream and discover all the amazing things that God has for us," Myles says. In her work as a coach in this area, Myles has proven that we carry this deep-seated fear for years, and it's not until this burden is lifted that we can soar and live life freely. "Being crippled by fear is dysfunctional at its very root," says the busy wife and mother, who stepped out on faith and left what was considered a set-for-life corporate position to own her dreams and fulfill her purpose. In addition to her coaching practice, Myles founded the Sister Accord Foundation to promote the power of loving, trusting, and loyal relationships in transforming every aspect of the lives of girls and women. She also authored *The Sister Accord: 51 Ways to Love Your Sister*. When asked what starts the process of healing, Myles says without hesitation, "Understanding where your fear originated and what triggers it so you can shut it down."

POWER POINT

Don't own your challenges. They've only come for a season, one that will add to your growth, so keep moving boldly in the direction of your dreams!

Fear is like a drug, and if we're not careful, we can become addicted to it, dare not to dream, and accept a space of being mentally crippled as our due, or interpret stagnation as being "safe." I know the former firsthand. As a young girl, I was always outspoken and took every opportunity to express whatever was on my mind, firmly believing that I had a right to do so. In an age when "children should be seen and not heard," this was a problem, and my elders told me that because of my verbal disobedience I would not live to reach age fifty, and I believed them. Living with this burden of fear impacted my life and some of my most critical decisions. In fact, once I turned fifty, I had no script, no dreams to discover, just a blank page because I never thought I'd see it. Moreover, this belief even impacted my finances, and I used a lot of my retirement funds to send our last child to the private university of her desires because I believed that I'd never live to use the money for its intended purpose. When I turned fifty, I said, "And now what?" Everybody expected me to have a big birthday party and I didn't want one. I was like a fish out of water. I went to Oprah's fiftieth celebration at Harpo Studios and had such a great time that I decided that was enough celebration for everyone! Understand that I didn't lack for birthday parties growing up as my mother threw birthday parties for me everywhere from our home to swanky restaurants and grandiose destinations with larger-than-life gifts and surprises, like the time she flew in with a stuffed monkey from Sammy Davis Jr. that was so big it had to have its own seat on the plane! So here I am at age fifty, and when I finally came to grips with the fact that "you're not going anywhere till God gets ready," I also came to understand that my grandmother did her best in helping my mother bring up an outspoken child by using the Old Testament scripture of "Honor thy father and thy mother that thy days may be long" as a yardstick to do so. And though I don't condone disrespectfulness in children—or adults, for that matter—and accept that the price I paid was both daunting and measurable, the wisdom that accompanied it is invaluable. I also took accountability for accepting this fear as a verdict and allowing it to halt the fearless woman in me who, upon graduation from high school, told her parents that she wouldn't need the money they had saved for her to go to college to do what she was going to do. I couldn't articulate back then why I felt so empowered in using my voice, but years later, when I became a speaker and began to do television, I understood it ever so clearly. When I became beauty director at *Essence* magazine, I also understood why, growing up, I had such an insatiable desire for storytelling and dolls, which I styled and created story lines around until age fourteen, because it was my *internship* to the role of working with the "living dolls" I'd be putting on the pages of the magazine and on the cover to affirm our beauty, all shades, shapes, and sizes.

Truth is, when you get a divine assignment, it's fully packaged—that's why you're not supposed to be anxious or fearful, because God didn't just give you the gift. That would be like giving a child an inheritance without giving her the lessons on what to do with it and how to grow it. He packaged your gift to take you from level to level. It's when we're fearful that we get stuck and allow people to box us in and limit our lives. "Then we get in these reality boxes that we didn't dream of and wonder why we feel stunted or stifled," says Lake, who fearlessly partnered with a sister-friend and created a successful interior design business and, in addition to *Paternity Court*, hosted *Spice Up My Kitchen* on HGTV.

66 "There is no greater agony than bearing an untold story inside of you."
—Dr. Maya Angelou

I've learned that fear can be a great obstacle if you *let* it, but you must lead with the greatness that lies in you and refuse to surrender. As we mature, we learn to overcome old fears, but if we're not grounded, new fears can take their place, both positive—those that compel you to master something "afraid," like pursuing a longed-for career choice or a passion—or the negative kind of fear that can hold you back, like being terrified to speak up and express yourself or try something new. We fear success as much as we fear failure when both represent opportunities to grow. As for the latter, I especially say don't fear failure, as some of the best people I know have failed their way to the top. What made them winners is they kept on taking the tests and pursuing the challenges until they got it great—not good but *great*! There's a success element to failure, and what I say is if you're going to fail, you ought to fail well, and the way to do that is to learn from your errors and let these experiences teach you what to do and what not to do on the way to accomplishment. Keep in mind, things don't always happen to you; they also happen *for* you. Oftentimes your purpose is on the other side of your pain or your biggest challenge. In fact, pain and challenge have provoked many into their purpose. How many of us have been on jobs where we were devalued, disrespected, and pushed to the point where we said "enough" and finally stepped out on faith to do what we'd been putting off for a check? "I believe there is an empire within each of us as there's a way to turn pain, purpose, and passions into profit by learning how to create a life doing what you do best," Lake points out. My sister, Candace, loves people, and her gift is one of helping others. Right after high school she had her own beauty salon, and it was a destination for artistic dos. The salon stayed full of women and children, and I know they came as much for a great hairstyle as they did for the nurturing experience she provided. While enjoying this success, she was in a relationship that turned abusive. Recognizing that love doesn't hurt, she ended it and turned this challenge into a win by taking ownership of her life, authoring her first book, *Ice: Careful Don't Burn Yourself* (a thriller that tells the story of a young girl whose life is forever altered by the choices she makes), and today, as a happily married mom of two, counsels young women on domestic violence. Do you think that was a coincidence? No! "Purpose is about developing the lens through which we see life and asking yourself, 'How can I be purposeful in it? How can I make it better?'" Lake concludes.

Define what's valuable to you. Don't allow others to live their lives vicariously through you. You're not a chauffeur to someone else's dreams.

Mikki-ism

There's a first-time fear for everything, but I've learned to encourage myself in my most fearful and broken moments when I am at the brink of giving up with an affirmation that says: "You're just the girl for the challenge, and if God brought you to it, He'll bring you through it!" What's critical to your every day is to keep your inner dialogue doubt-free and faith-forward. Agree to put the stronghold of fear and insecurity on lockdown and be fearless; you weren't created to be crippled by these emotions, so don't manufacture them. Don't shrink back; step forward! Learn to encourage yourself and be audacious. Own that you are fine, fierce, and focused on all things good. Recognize that you were created for the best, across the board, in life, in love, your career, whatever it is that concerns you, and trust God's promises and His training without measure. Understand, too, that no one else gets to decide what's best for you; that's called giving your power away, and you don't want to be guilty of that. I remember the days when I used to "go along to get along," afraid to displease anyone, and everybody was happy except me. Then one day I was on an *Essence* cover shoot working with two difficult celebrities, and wouldn't you know it, things became so tense, it was really a question of "you're darned if you do and you're darned if you don't," and I decided if I'm going to be the "fall gal," then I was through compromising. As a result, the subjects walked out and I didn't get the cover shot (which could have been disastrous), and that's when I learned that fear serves no purpose other than to hold you back. I learned to accept responsibility, not blame, and there is a difference. When you accept responsibility, you can stand behind your decisions whether others agree with you or not, *and* you accept the same degree of responsibility whether you are proven right *or* wrong. When you accept blame, you only concede guilt, and as a result your confidence and your capabilities will suffer and ultimately you will become a fearful follower, not a leader. Some of us have a lifelong legacy of fear that we need to outgrow so we can come into our divine inheritance as the leaders we were created to be. The Word has it that God didn't give us the spirit of fear but of power, and there's no sense in being gifted with it if you don't have the tenacity to work it!

Don't come to the "party" after everything's put away. Get out of your own way! Dream big, be bold!

Mikki-ism

If fear has you hesitant to seize your dreams and fulfill your purpose, then I need to tell you you're afraid of the wrong thing. You ought to be afraid of not being who God says you are and accomplishing what He has gifted you to do. You ought to be afraid of making provisions for your insecurities, and you need to put that fear on lockdown and say, "I'm not the one!" Avow that you were designed unto a purpose and refuse to get in the way. Moving forward, whenever and wherever fear creeps and no matter where it originates from, you must continue to realize that you can't use it and the solution lies not in blaming the cause but in releasing it and refuting its triggers so you can discover the transformative power that lies within you. Again, you must not manufacture fear. Experts tell us that half the things we worry about never happen. How many yesterdays and todays have you sacrificed living in fear of an imaginary tomorrow that isn't designed for your good? Don't let self-imposed fear cause you to live in the shadow of your own life and who you were created to be. Determine that you're going to possess the kind of faith that silences all fears and objections, and allow the Giver of life to propel you forward. According to Myles and other experts, there's a spiritual and physiological peace to this that impacts your well-being, so get with it. Decide today to develop the plan that moves you from where you are to where you desire to be. Start by identifying that which burns in your heart, and know that it's what you have been created to do. Myles confirms this is as simple as beginning to visualize how it will show up and how others will experience it. From there it's about creating a prioritized plan to bring it to life because vision without execution is simply hallucination. So be strategic in walking out your purpose by planning it out through manageable components that will allow you to bring it to fulfillment, and then commit to staying on track with it. This is the time to turn to your celebration circle as they will propel and support you on the journey. You'll also want to enlist mentors who can advise and tour you through the process as well. Most of all, establish your "brand advocates," people who can speak for you and help move you to the next level.

The Check-Out

If you're looking to identify your purpose and blaze a trail, check out the following reads:

Abundance Now, by Lisa Nichols

Exponential Living: Stop Spending 100% of Your Time on 10% of Who You Are, by Sheri Riley

Find Your Fierce: Answering Your Soul's Call to Purpose, Power & Profit, by Nicole Roberts Jones

Act Like a Success, Think Like a Success: Discovering Your Gift and the Way to Life's Riches, by Steve Harvey

---

66 **N**o matter the picture in which you find yourself, write your own script. Dream, but be present where you are, right now. Embrace the perfect now. See. Hear. Smell. Taste. Don't wait, breathe."

—Alfre Woodard, actress, producer, political activist

It's about blazing a trail instead of taking the road well traveled.

Mikki-ism

Know that thriving on the path of self-discovery is more than a notion or the temporary euphoria that comes from a spa vacation, and there's a distinct difference between dreaming and *daydreaming*. The former is essential; the latter is for children. You don't want a "virtual reality"; you deserve to have the real thing. You have the power to bring your dreams to life, free yourself from erroneous underlying assumptions, and make those all-important self-discoveries—you just have to learn how to use them—so don't wander in the wilderness of doubt or hesitation. I believe there are many facets that lie inside each of us, and we owe it to ourselves to experience them all. I learned that I have an adventurous spirit, and I love exploring it. I took up white-water rafting between the mountains in West Virginia and fell in love with the

Notes to Self...

2

Skin: It's a New Day

Who doesn't want to be in the glow? I love how brown skin looks post a well-rested vacation when it's fresh, radiant, and dewy! The good news is nowadays this kind of vitality doesn't require a boarding pass to achieve because the promise of great skin is surer than ever with the right practices and today's game-changing ingredients, pro treatments, and DIY tools. Now, this doesn't mean that we can toss aside such factors as a healthy lifestyle, a targeted skin care regimen, and a diet full of antioxidants and plant-based foods, but when coupled with supercharging efforts, getting there now is a lot more direct.

Skin GPS

Multiple factors come into play and contribute to the look and texture of your skin. In fact, there's a long-running checklist that forms your skin's current profile with factors that range from genetics to the effects of sun damage, smoking, and allergens, to hyperpigmentation, acne, the aging process, improper care, sleep deprivation, even how you wear your hair or press your cell phone (which has more bacteria than a toilet seat!) against your face—all of these have a visible impact. This is why I say when it comes to possessing great skin, a gal's best strategy is one of informed defense rather than damage control. According to Dr. Ro, author of *Lose Your Final 15: Dr. Ro's Plan to Eat 15 Servings a Day and Lose 15 Pounds at a Time*, changing lives 15 pounds at a time, nurturing your skin calls for a targeted diet that includes copious amounts of colorful vegetables and fruits. "These are foods whose pigments contain antioxidants and phytochemicals that protect our skin and make it youthful, dewy, and supple," says the award-winning health journalist and nutrition coach for *The Dr. Oz Show*. Dr. Ro, who's known for her easy-to-apply advice for women and families, also encourages us to put down the sugary drinks and replace them with lots of water because, as she says, "sugar is highly inflammatory to the skin and it causes acne."

There's no question, you need to deeply understand the skin you're in, how and what it responds to, and what keeps it fresh and healthy year-round, and it's more than just "cleanse, tone, and moisturize." Today's strategy is one of "cleanse, treat, and protect," and the objective of "tone" has morphed into such treatment practices as microdermabrasion, chemical peels, mesotherapy, and pore-perfecting gadgets that encourage cell turnover (which slows down around age twenty-five), stimulate collagen, and help reveal your best skin. "The entire future of skin care is trending as quickly as the Apple iPhone," says celebrity aesthetician Mamie McDonald. At her busy NYC destination, Skin by Mamie, McDonald cites the types of treatment that African American women want and notes that they have changed in the last five years from just wanting their skin to look clean, plump, soft, and beautiful to include more targeted procedures involving injectables like Botox and fillers. "Black women are much more concerned about their appearance, and I'm not talking women age forty-five and up, I'm talking about the millennials," says McDonald. "I'm doing more procedures on skin of color than I would have previously done, and it's driven by my patients' requests."

"They're pushing the envelope," concurs NYC dermatologist Rose-marie Ingleton, citing Botox to address expression lines and fillers to enhance facial volume as being in big demand. From where I sit, everyone is involved in next-level care and highly engaged in the age-defying game, and it's never too early to start.

The Influencers

You + aesthetician + dermatologist all play a role in achieving your best skin. Forget any notion that aestheticians and the services they provide are a luxury or that you don't need to see a dermatologist unless something is wrong. Look at it this way: partnering with both is an investment in your beauty that has great benefits. In fact, nowadays you'll find aestheticians and dermatologists working out of the same facility. "In my practice, I have a medical aesthetician who does supplementary procedures like a facial, and less-risky processes that I supervise," Dr. Ingleton explains. Another advantage to be found in environments like this is the quality of the equipment is more advanced than at a spa, and with the dermatologist supervising the settings, "the aesthetician can do more aggressive procedures," she adds. I'm big on at-home maintenance, but if you want to possess skin that glows year-round, it's best to partner with an aesthetician for the proper diagnosis, customized facials, and specific services like microdermabrasion that have been determined to keep your skin at its best. You'll want to see a dermatologist for annual (face and body) checkups and prescription-treatment products, Botox, fillers, ultrasound-based Ultherapy, or laser treatments and to address skin care concerns like discoloration, acne, eczema, flesh moles, rashes, and allergic reactions, as well as facial hair removal, hair loss, or any nail disorders. Where there are concerns, always be sure to schedule an appointment sooner rather than later because patience *isn't* a virtue when there's cause for concern. More often than not, the longer you wait to have it checked out, the more damage control will be required of the expert you see, lessening your chances for optimal results.

To find a dermatologist in your area, go to the website of the National Medical Association (NMA), an organization that promotes the interests of physicians and patients of African descent, at www.nmanet.org, and see the "physician locator" for a doctor in your area; you can consult the state and local society listings on this website as well. If further assistance is needed, you can contact the NMA directly at 1-202-347-1895, where a live representative will help you locate a derm by specialty.

The Naked Truth

Great skin care begins with consulting an aesthetician to understand your skin's basic ID. Here's a spot check to give you an indication:

- **Dry:** Taut, has an ashy cast, feels itchy, shows tiny surface lines.
- **Oily:** Shiny, produces more sebum than average, feels slick, prone to breakouts, has large pores, can experience acne.
- **Combination:** Oily in the T-zone (forehead, nose, and chin), dry on the sides, breaks out occasionally.
- **Sensitive:** Easily irritated, itchy, often dry, has a tendency to be blotchy.

POWER POINT

The intrinsic aging process begins in our twenties, though it may not be apparent for decades. What's key is how well you play defense in the area of self-care.

Primed for Greatness

On a most basic level, establishing a skin care regimen that nurtures your skin, keeping it healthy by proper cell turnover and protecting it from the damaging rays of the sun, is of prime importance. "Your daily skin care routine has the most impact, so you must have a routine that you are consistently doing that includes cleansing, using sun protection, and applying something nutritious on your skin every day," Ingleton says. Here it's not about shopping labels or assuming that an expensive product pick is a guaranteed option, but shopping with the kind of savvy that considers both your skin type as well as your lifestyle, which also impacts how your skin looks and behaves. Quite honestly, I like fabulous packaging and what's trending like the next girl, but I caution you to beware of prioritizing design elements, marketing promises, and enticing buzzwords over your skin type and what it requires. For example, if you've got dry, sensitive skin, you're not the gal who needs an astringent, no matter how savvily it's packaged or billed, and you're probably not a candidate for a lot of the trending products with "active" ingredients (e.g., glycolic acid pads) no matter how many social media posts they get! When shopping for products, take your cues from reliable sources with product and ingredient knowledge as what's popular or performs for someone in your circle may not work for you. Take the category of sun-protection products. What may be invisible on someone who's fairer than you may look gray on your rich brown skin tone, so it pays to be wise and shop with your skin top of mind. My number one skin commandment is still "Know thyself and own the skin you're in."

We're not getting any more
hours in the day, so don't
underestimate the power of great
skin care. It's the best staycation
going for your beauty!

Mikki-ism

About Face

In terms of your lifestyle, the amount of rest you get (or not), the environment you work in, and the time you have to devote to the care of your skin, even with your travel schedule, is worth assessing. According to McDonald, one of many who cites our fast-paced lifestyle as a contributor to the lack of optimal skin health, reports an increase in her treatment practice of skin damaged from air travel. "Air travel saps the life out of your skin. There's only 30 percent moisture in the cabin of an airplane (and it's recirculated at that). It dries out the skin, and as a result I'm addressing the flare-up of tiny bumps, rashes, and skin so dehydrated that it's almost like a sunburn," she says. As someone who goes "wheels up" every week sometimes, I can relate. My defense is to skip caffeinated beverages (also dehydrating) and wear a moisturizer that contains hyaluronic acid, as this super juicy ingredient holds up to a thousand times its weight in water; on long-haul flights, I reapply it every ninety minutes. I also use sunscreen, as UV rays are more intense at higher altitudes and I'm usually in a window seat. Go figure! All this and more have caused me to think about what impacts great skin and the role we play in it.

Sleeping Beauty

A lot of us are big on work and short on sleep, and yet sleep is the time when skin repairs itself, essentially making it one of the best treatments we have access to on a daily basis. Failing to get adequate sleep results in inflammation of the skin and also affects the immune system. As McDonald notes, when this is the case, anything that lies dormant will flare up. I know if my schedule calls for repeated nights where I have to "sleep fast" (my interpretation of reduced sleep time), eczema resurfaces on my back *and* my complexion looks dull and off duty! In a ground-breaking study commissioned by Estée Lauder with University Hospitals Case Medical Center, the primary affiliate of Case Western Reserve University School of Medicine, lack of sleep can accelerate signs of skin aging, and women who typically slept less than five hours had more fine lines, uneven pigmentation, and sagging slackening of skin. Additionally, the results indicated that poor-quality sleep can slow skin's natural repair processes. I don't blame a gal who puts her best foot forward at work and in life, but it's best to strike a balance and, along with topical care, go to bed so you can look your best and not hasten the aging process. In addition, don't forgo protecting your skin before retiring, as this will cost you, too. If you come home too tired to wash the day off your face and hit your pillow with pollutants in tow, your skin will give evidence with clogged pores. The same holds true if you fail to tie your hair up at night and protect your skin from the airborne impurities as well as the hair products in your do. McDonald cites the big turn to natural hair and many of the ingredients in the products used as a call for awareness and consistent preventive measures for the skin. "Most of the leave-in care products contain glycerin or shea butter or some kind of oil, and once any of these come in contact with your skin, breakouts will occur because the skin cannot breathe," says the busy aesthetician, who keeps celebs like Tasha Smith and TV personality Tai Beauchamp in the glow. "We're constantly on a quest to find that product that's going to make our hair look nice and shiny, and we're not thinking about what products are going to cause an effect on my skin," Ingleton states. Ingleton, who works a chic natural herself, sighs that the popular use of shea butters and castor oil are a huge red flag "because along with the use of these products, which are lovely and wonderful, I'm seeing more acne." Factors like these, along with the given that most of us cannot wash our hair every day, are why protecting our skin at night is a must. Seeing how the realities of modern life can play a role in the health of your skin, I say be more proactive by controlling what's in your power.

AFFIRMATION

"I know who I am, and I've always been
comfortable in my own skin."

—Ledisi, singer, songwriter, actress

Fresh Start

Cherish your beautiful brown skin like you would that of a newborn. You moms know what I'm talking about because you pay close attention to your baby's skin and incorporate what is essentially a care regimen to keep their skin clean, hydrated, and protected. Your skin deserves the same with a heightened approach in that you should look to products that offer both short- and long-term benefits. In determining your best strategy, know that cleansing twice a day, with the most effective cleanser for your skin type to remove dead skin cells and impurities, is the backbone of any successful care routine. From there, it's about treating and protecting your skin with performance-driven products and practices that reveal your best skin and keep it in the glow.

When it comes to skin care picks, I'm not of the school of thought that "one size serves all." I like a targeted approach.

Mikki-ism

Cleanse

Clean Sweep

We're all thrilled by the next new thing, but a lot of beauty basics remain in effect among the pros. What's changed are the next-level formulations and new-era ingredients that give you more bang for your buck than those of yesteryear. For my normal/combination skin, I rely on a tech-savvy creamy foaming wash that can also double as a mask when I need it. It's on call most of the year as it effectively addresses my sensitivity while checking my oil and not parching my dry areas. In the depths of summer, I use an enzymatic gel cleanser that is more efficient as we all get a little oilier at this time of the year. I also deep-clean weekly, as professionally advised, with an oscillating facial cleansing brush to slough off dead skin cells (see "Oscillating Brushes," under "Game Changers" page 97). In navigating your best cleanser(s) and the proper routine, consult the experts; don't self-assess. A licensed aesthetician, a dermatologist, or at least a *knowledgeable* salesperson is invaluable as he or she can (A) assess your skin type and (B) identify your best care strategy.

If your skin is oily, an oil-free foaming cleanser that checks oil without stripping your skin is advised. "It's crucial to avoid being squeaky-clean because your natural oils are there to protect your skin," says NYC dermatologist Dr. Fran Cook-Bolden. Depending on your needs, a cleanser containing salicylic or glycolic acid may be suggested to help prevent breakouts. Dry skin dictates a mild, hydrating, creamy cleanser, some of which are nonfoaming with milder surfactants and moisturizers or nourishing oil-based cleansers that dissolve makeup as a bonus. All cleanse without drying, while combination skin can call for a gel, or creamy cleansers that foam, or a bar specifically designed to thoroughly clean without stimulating oil production or clogging pores. If you're acne-prone, cleansers containing salicylic acid or benzoyl peroxide, both of which deep-clean and reduce blemishes, are still the go-to choices. There are also those that contain kaolin clay or charcoal to draw out impurities. Here, it's about using a formula that's effective enough to deep-clean without causing irritation that can make your acne flare up. For women of color with acne-prone skin, consulting a dermatologist is crucial for proper treatment—from cleansing to care—to prevent post-inflammatory hyperpigmentation. For sensitive skin, look to those products that have the least amount of preservatives and are fragrance-free (which means they can contain a masking scent), dermatologist-tested, moisturizing, and extremely gentle. Depending on your degree of sensitivity, you may require a soapless cleanser or a micellar water cleanser (particularly if your skin is dry), which is very gentle and hydrating.

Morning Shift

Begin each day with your appropriate cleanser as step number one for soft, fresh skin. Coming clean with the right formulation preps your skin and allows the ingredients in your treatment picks to take effect.

- Think of cleansing your skin as the important treatment practice that it is, and start your approach by making sure

to use warm or lukewarm water, as hot water can dehydrate
your skin.

◉ Rinse thoroughly—not excessively. Again, squeaky-clean is
the antithesis of TLC.

◉ Keep in mind that all skin types like to be "babied," so in
drying your skin, pat—don't rub!

◉ Change face towels daily and use fragrance-free detergents
when laundering.

Night Watch

Waking up with glowing skin has everything to do with what you do
before hitting the pillows, and no matter how tired you are, you'll want
to do yourself a few favors before you "run out of gas."

◉ Make time to cleanse off the day: everything from pollutants
to makeup have gone along for the ride on your daily grind,
so don't even think about sleeping with these "frenemies"!
Depending on your skin type, reach for a good milky or
emollient cleanser that removes everything before washing
your face. If you wear long-wearing eye makeup formulas, I
suggest using a makeup remover made specifically for these
resistant formulas to prevent rubbing this delicate area and
causing any irritation. Cotton pads or loose cotton that
can be purchased by the roll are most effective for use in
removing makeup, as they are the most absorbent. Bottom
line: even if you're not a makeup wearer, use an effective
cleanser or cleansing wipe to be sure you come clean.

⦿ As often as is appropriate for your skin, give it the extra help it needs and slough off those lingering dead skin cells that don't want to relinquish their position once you're in your thirties with a good oscillating facial brush and a cleanser *or* a chemical exfoliant that contains fruit enzymes or chemical acids. You can also use a manual facial exfoliator if professionally approved should you like a hands-on experience, but do exfoliate with care. Physically abrasive products can cause unnecessary irritation. Know that if you're already using retinol on your skin, most experts advise against an additional exfoliating step as your skin is already experiencing fast cell turnover.

⦿ Prep for the repair process that happens while you sleep by applying a hydrating eye cream and a suitable treatment to address your skin and boost radiance.

⦿ You'll get extra credit by way of gorgeous skin if you use a humidifier to keep your skin moist and supple in the winter *and* be sure to sleep on a silk pillowcase as cotton cases zap moisture.

Lighten Up

When warmer temps usher themselves in, be "beauty ready." Warm weather signals it's time to switch to lighter skin care formulations and tweak your regimen to prevent clogged pores and makeup breakup. Again, everyone tends to be somewhat oilier when the heat and humidity set in, and this may call for a change in your routine and your maintenance products, starting with your cleanser, especially if minor breakouts begin to occur. You might even need to rest your favorite moisturizing cream for a lighter lotion formula, with SPF of course. You may also need to add a product that checks oil and a primer to keep your makeup intact if you're not already incorporating one as part of your regimen. You won't have to put your serum on hold, though, as they're lightweight and designed to penetrate into the skin immediately. Talk about complexion perfection.

---

66 If you're going to strip your skin, you better nourish it, or by the time you're forty-five, you're going to look ninety!"

—Mamie McDonald, aesthetician

Treat

Nurturing your skin by layering the minimal amount of products with the most concentrated ingredients is *the* strategic move now. In keeping with this modern-day approach, serums have become one of the superstars of the day for delivering high-performance ingredients directly into the skin to address everything from hydration to hyperpigmentation. "It's like the saying 'There's an app for that.' I tell my clients, 'There's a serum for that,'" says McDonald. Designed to be the first layer of care after cleansing, serums deliver active ingredients, antioxidants, and vitamins deeper into the skin in high concentrations most efficiently because of their smaller molecules, making them top contenders for every skin type as they are light and quickly absorbed. Among the many benefits the pros rely on them for are to hydrate, improve texture, plump, brighten, repair, regulate oil production, combat aging, and improve the efficacy of other skin care products in a regimen. Traditional serums are water-based, but there are many that are also oil-based. Facial oils are also a go-to pick for hydration, nutrition, and renewal as they contain beneficial plant oils. They're fine for all skin types with the exception of those who are acne-prone. They are also designed to be used post cleansing while skin is still warm and moist prior to your moisturizer to keep vital hydration locked in. During the cold seasons, my skin loves argan oil, which I use under a moisturizer with hyaluronic acid to seal in moisture, plump, and boost a summerlike radiance. With these technologically driven treatments, a little goes a long way, so think of massaging in a pea-size amount prior to applying your moisturizer.

Protect

When I first started reporting, many brown-skin beauties and companies alike took for granted that the melanin in our skin was a natural defense that protected us from the aging effects of the sun and kept us out of harm's way when it came to skin cancer. But times have changed, and despite the fact that melanin does offer us *some* protection, experts strongly advise us to shield ourselves on a daily basis as part of a wise care strategy year-round. "I'm sorry to tell you Black does crack and the best treatment for African American women is to avoid ultraviolet rays from the sun, which is responsible for 70 percent of visible aging," says Beverly Hills dermatologist and skin care specialist Dr. Susan Evans, who stands on the fact that sunscreen is imperative. In her NYC office, Dr. Fran Cook-Bolden is also a proponent of sun protection: "The ozone is continuing to narrow, and our melanin is not protecting us enough, we're wrinkling at an earlier age, we're seeing sun damage and skin cancer increase," she shared. To protect yourself, maintain an even tone, and guard against damaging UV rays, which can break down collagen in the skin, which results in a loss of fullness and accelerated aging, use an SPF (sun protection factor) of 30 and apply it from your hairline to your chest.

Think of it as an investment pick and find a formula that you love and use it religiously. On the face, you'll want to avoid any pore-clogging ingredients like cocoa butter and coconut oil; however, if oils are your thing, technology has come to the rescue, so you can hydrate, glow, and protect with products like L'Oréal Paris Age Perfect Hydra-Nutrition Facial Oil SPF 30, which is formulated with essential oils. Those of us with deeper skin tones need to save face and steer clear of those chalky formulas that leave behind a white cast due to titanium dioxide and instead look to those that are sheer on us. Here again, choosing a product means considering your needs and desires as well as your skin type and, where necessary, looking at its purpose from a lifestyle perspective. For example, for wear under foundation, a seamless formula that protects and hydrates is a basic (pros advise the use of sunscreen even if your foundation of choice contains SPF, as this should be viewed as an added benefit, not a replacement for full protection). You'll also find products with an SPF that have treatment benefits and contain ingredients to improve the texture of your skin. A day at the beach or extended outdoor activities call for a product designed to resist water and sweat, usually a lotion or cream formulation, with a higher SPF, and it should be applied liberally and often (every two hours). To protect an exposed scalp due to a shaved head, cornrows, or flat twists, use a gel with an SPF of 30 to protect this often-overlooked area from burning. Know that if you use skin care products containing alpha hydroxy acids or retinol, your skin will be more photosensitive, so be sure to apply sunscreen *before* makeup, and allow time for it to dry thoroughly. Make sure to also use an SPF of at least 15 on the lips, whether you wear lipstick or not, and reapply frequently, as lips do burn.

Protecting our skin is an essential component to maintaining pretty brown skin, especially if you're trying to micromanage uneven pigmentation, because the sun activates melanin production, making our efforts at fading dark spots or hyperpigmented areas totally in vain.

Glamour in the Sun

I find looking fab at the beach is a quite chic game of show-and-tell and always requires a little beauty navigation. First things first: before you attempt to put one pedicured toe in the sand, please limit your exposure between the hours of ten and two, when the sun's rays are the strongest. Now, that being said, I suggest getting an ultrachic hat to protect your skin (and your hair, especially if you have color). Wherever you're headed, keep the look "barely there and glowy"—translation: facial moisturizer with SPF 30; groomed brows set with clear mascara; gold-flecked body oil with sunscreen, which is a gorgeous way to get your glow on; and a shimmery lip balm with an SPF of 15. Perfection!

POWER POINT

A woman's skin changes throughout her lifetime. This calls for a real strategy to keep skin on course and healthy. Don't second-guess this; consult a pro, as the risk of damage for skin of color is far too great.

Game Changers

Scoring and maintaining your best skin is at your fingertips with non-invasive treatments, pro procedures, next-level ingredients, and modern DIY devices that target our biggest concerns. Welcome to the new generation of beauty boosters! According to Dr. Rosemarie Ingleton, a woman who's known for her skin-renewing practices, "to achieve radiance, it's all about skin renewal, and you get this when you constantly renew your skin cells. We're taking advantage of fruit acids, exfoliating gadgets to get a deeper clean, microdermabrasion, and chemical peels—all of which help to remove dead cells and bring fresh cells to the surface."

Facials

Facials are still the favored choice for soft, clean, rejuvenated skin. The art of today's facials is in the assessment, and this again is where a great aesthetician is key. Trends come and go, and while there are all kinds of facials, the best treatment is one that has been customized for you. It's best then to partner with an aesthetician and allow her to determine what type of facial your skin needs and how often. I don't quite understand how someone can call a spa or a skin care salon and book something on the menu without knowing what her needs are, which is why I suggest booking an hour with the aesthetician simply for a "facial." Once your skin is analyzed, a basic facial will include a massage to stimulate circulation (which alone is worth the entire session) under a mist of comfortably hot steam; any necessary extractions will then take place, followed by a mask suitable for your complexion. Having said as much, here is a checklist of those facials that give us the most mileage when properly matched to skin type and when combined with an appropriate at-home care regimen:

Deep-cleansing/Purifying: A basic treatment suitable for most skin types, but especially beneficial for those with oily/combination skin. It removes impurities and nourishes the skin, leaving it soft and smooth.

Oxygen: For all skin types, it especially revitalizes dull, dehydrated skin with the addition of pure oxygen to nourish the cells, increase collagen production, and bring about a glow.

Vitamin C: A powerful antioxidant, vitamin C removes dead skin cells, imparts brightness, and creates radiant, new skin—a boost for all skin types.

Hydrating: Aimed at nurturing dry or mature skin or skin dehydrated by environmental factors, this treatment stimulates circulation, softens, and replenishes moisture.

Sheet Masks

Billed as one-sheet wonders, sheet masks are the new skin-salvation picks for at-home use. Composed of cotton or fiber that is cut in the shape of one's face, they come presoaked with revitalizing ingredients like peptides, antioxidants, niacinamide, amino acids, and other patented ingredients to boost radiance, hydrate, tighten, and revive skin in the time it takes to enjoy your favorite latte. I love them in between facials, especially when air travel has zapped the life out of my skin and I need to appear looking fresh and can't catch my zzz's (oxymoronic, right?). While they don't take the place of a professional mask, they do drive powerful ingredients into your skin, deliver instant gratification, don't require rinsing, and can be found at all price points. There are also eye masks to eliminate puffiness and soften fine lines, as well as sheet masks for your feet that exfoliate dead skin and soften.

Touch-Up Masks

When it comes to at-home products, I'm your original "test girl" (you didn't think I was going to refer to myself as a guinea pig did you?—not!) as I'm forever testing new offerings, much to the dismay of my skin care team. Masks have come a long way from the messy, underwhelming picks they used to be, and thanks to technology, they're now like a "doc in a box" on call when you need them. They're also a nurturing way to be good to the Queen who lies in you. I call them touch-up masks, though, because far be it from Yours Truly to be less than honest with you, so know that nothing can replace a professional facial. That being said, there's a mask to suit every skin type and every purpose, and picks are at the ready to lift impurities, hydrate, tighten, brighten, and more. Here are some "fixers" for serving great face:

Goal: Detox by drawing out impurities, unclog pores.
Try: GlamGlow Supermud Clearing Treatment, Kiehl's Rare

Earth Deep Pore Cleansing Mask, Philosophy Purity Made Simple Pore Extractor Exfoliating Clay Mask.

Goal: Hydrate, soothe, refresh, renew.
Try: Fresh Rose Face Mask, Dior Hydra Life Beauty Awakening Rehydrating Mask, Clinique Moisture Surge Overnight Mask.

Goal: Firm/tighten, plump, glow.
Try: Peter Thomas Roth 24K Gold Pure Luxury Lift & Firm Mask, Clarins Extra-Firming Mask, L'Oréal Revitalift Triple Power Intensive Overnight Mask.

Goal: Brighten, event-prep.
Try: Bliss Triple Oxygen Instant Energizing Foaming Mask, Dr. Brandt Oxygen Facial Flash Recovery Mask, Fresh Vitamin Nectar Vibrancy-Boosting Face Mask.

Oscillating Brushes

Rotary brushes are unbeatable for their sonic cleansing and exfoliating capabilities, which clean out pores in minutes. If the results of soft, ultra-buffed skin weren't enough, another benefit of these DIY investment-worthy picks is how well your skin care products penetrate post use. This "power tool" has become my Sunday night special, where I put the brush to work with a creamy cleanser (designed for use with the brush), followed by a hydrating mask and then my serum to nourish my skin overnight. Come Monday morning, my skin always looks as if I've had a great getaway! If you're a devotee, however, know that experts do caution against being overly zealous with this increasingly popular cleansing tool. "Be sure to only use a cleansing brush a maximum of three times a week, with twenty-four to forty-eight hours in between," McDonald says. You should also use it with a suitable cleanser and never pair it with an exfoliating (granular) cleanser as the brush itself exfoliates. McDonald, who also keeps celebs like Angela Bassett and Iman camera-ready, advises caring for your brush meticulously. "Make sure that you wash the brush head immediately and at least once a week put it in the microwave for ten seconds to kill the active bacteria that grows from the moisture in your bathroom. Put it in Saran wrap and keep it in your refrigerator until the next time you use it." A good quality oscillating facial brush ranges in price from just under $30 to more than $250.

Microdermabrasion

This skin-renewing treatment, where aluminum oxide crystals are gently sprayed onto the face, neck, and chest and then lightly sucked away with a vacuum along with your dead cells, is performed by both dermatologists and aestheticians. It leaves skin baby-soft and smooth, improves tone and texture irregularities, softens fine lines, and increases collagen production. It's worth noting that receiving the procedure in a dermatologist's office will differ from that available in a salon or spa because the machines offered to doctors have more intense settings than those offered to aestheticians. Nowadays most experts favor a form of combination therapy to address our top concerns such as monthly facials and microdermabrasion or mild chemical peels and a cocktail of supernutrients delivered deep into the skin. At Skin by Mamie, where every treatment process is customized, McDonald follows my microdermabrasion treatments with a mask based on my skin condition, be it with active ingredients such as lactic acid to speed cell renewal and ramp up radiance or hyaluronic acid and algae to boost hydration and reduce visible imperfections and hyperpigmentation. Post mask, vitamins A, C, and E are massaged directly onto my skin. An oxygen blast is also included via an oxygen tank to cool, nourish the cells, and enhance the glow. You think I could mimic this at home? Not! These are the kinds of insights and professional support that underscore the value of having a skin care expert as part of your temple-management team, as discussed in the previous chapter. Microdermabrasion costs anywhere from $100 to $200 on average and requires no downtime; side effects are minimal but can include skin tightness and temporary sun sensitivity.

Chemical Peels

Complexion perfection is unlocked by today's chemical change agents used during a peel to exfoliate, unclog pores, address acne, improve dullness, and soften and smooth the skin. The big news is that today's peels are part of the unifying, all-together-now even-skin-tone procedures, and for us that's huge. During the resurfacing procedure, a chemical solution containing lactic, glycolic, or salicylic acid or fruit enzymes (which are the mildest) is applied to the skin, causing it to exfoliate and eventually peel off and reveal the fresh new layers that lie beneath. "Our skin is so sensitive and so reactive. It's been wonderful to explore some of the newer chemical peeling agents and products, and finding that we can use this on our skin as well," says Dr. Ingleton, who favors glycolic acid peels and salicylic acid peels. Such superficial or "lunchtime" peels, as they are called, are commonly used on skin of color, leaving it impressively smooth and radiant while causing an increase in collagen production. They also cause your skin care products to work better minus those dead skin cells that blocked their communication! Trichloroacetic acid (TCA), which is used for a medium-depth peel, penetrates the skin at a level that facilitates collagen renewal, reduces fine lines and hyperpigmentation, and decreases the appearance of large pores and moderate acne scarring. This type of peel should always be done by a medical professional and at the lowest percentage strength as it causes skin to peel and carries the risk of additional scarring for those with deeper skin tones. Another type of peel favored by dermatologists is the vitamin or retinoic acid peel, which consists of vitamin A. "I use the Vitalize Chemical Peel, which includes retinoic acid, but I also have relied on TCA peels in 10 percent or 15 percent and glycolic peels on 30 percent or lower and cautiously go up from there," says Dr. Sumayah Taliaferro, who, at her Atlanta, Georgia, practice, always errs on the side of observation and how a patient responds to initial treatment. Many dermatologists are also generating their own peel mixes to achieve multiple benefits to brighten and address hyperpigmentation. Chemical peels are applied using a brush or sponge to the skin and are accompanied by a stinging sensation depending on the chemical used. When considering any peel, be advised that most experts recommend only the mildest formulas for women of color, and strongly urge us to shun those that contain phenol, which lightens the skin and can be permanent. I also urge you to seek out a qualified professional who has experience administering peels on skin of color because you don't want to surrender your face to someone who simply got a certificate so he or she could hang up a sign advertising chemical peels! Given the fact that there's no rhyme or reason to the way melanin rushes in on our skin as a reaction to any and everything from an insect bite to a scrape, you don't want to risk getting a peel from inexperienced hands—the possible damage is just too great. This is also why you won't read about at-home peels in *EIC*. Enough said. Post treatment from a superficial peel, you can expect mild swelling and flaking but no downtime; medium-depth peels call for up to a week of downtime during which you can experience swelling and, again, peeling depending on the duration of the peel administered. Costs range from $200 for light chemical peels to as high as $1,000, depending on the expert performing the treatment.

Injectables

Botulinum toxin, commonly known as Botox (brand name), temporarily reduces frown lines, forehead creases, and crow's-feet by blocking nerve signals that cause muscles to contract, and cosmetic fillers like Restylane, Juvéderm, and Sculptra (to name a few) that improve volume and firmness, fill in fine lines, and promote collagen and elastin in the cheeks and other areas are the new "hot shots" for women of color. "For years, women of color didn't think that doing Botox was in the cards for them—they thought it was a procedure only white women did. Today my practice is heavily weighted with women of color who are coming for Botox *and* fillers just like any other woman," says Dr. Ingleton, whose lower Manhattan office has become a beauty destination. In the right hands, we can trust we'll get the results of our desires, and while we're not obsessed with aging, no one wants to look old, or tired for that matter! Uptown, Dr. Cook-Bolden is incorporating the use of fillers and Botox on African American women to enhance volume instead of using it to just fill in lines and address the active movement lines. More than just employing a process of "still and fill," Cook-Bolden takes into consideration both the short and long term and takes a "less is more" approach. "It's about building the skin back up and building integrity, instead of fillers that just fill in lines," she states. As is our mind-set for all things concerning our beauty, it's not about looking *done*—now when it comes to our hair, that's another story! This is true across the board for all ages and professions. "I'm undertreating. In fact, I call it 'Baby Botox,'" Ingleton states. Known for her attention to detail, she counts media professionals and celebrities among her clientele. "An actress will have Botox, but nobody can tell, not even the directors, but we both know when we look at her pictures, we can tell what was bothering her and how it totally fixes it, but not to the point where the rest of the world is saying, 'She got frozen,' or 'She got this or she got that.' That's been my forte because they'll get fired if they can't emote!" Ingleton says.

Neurotoxins or neuromuscular agents (generic names) are injected beneath the skin and into the muscle using a very fine needle. As the muscle stops contracting, the skin above it begins to smooth out, reducing or eliminating the appearance of fine lines. The results last anywhere from three to six months, though the benefits are said to be cumulative. Most people experience little if any discomfort as the areas of treatment are always numbed first with ice before the tiny injections begin. There is no downtime with the exception of flying, as doctors like Cook-

Bolden say you may not travel by airplane for two days after receiving Botox. Aside from being grounded, patients receive a small list of "dos & don'ts post treatment." Common side effects can include headache and bruising, the latter of which is preventable by applying ice. Costs range from $300 to $1,200, depending on how much is needed and who administers it.

Cosmetic fillers like Restylane and Juvéderm are composed of hyaluronic acid, which attaches to the skin and instantly adds volume. The procedure not only provides immediate results but also helps skin retain more moisture naturally. Results last from six to twelve months. Sculptra is made of poly-L-lactic acid, which stimulates collagen production, rebuilding lost facial volume and naturally lifting and filling sunken areas. Results from Sculptra can last up to two years. As with Botox injections, the skin is cleaned and numbed with ice prior, and the tiny injections of filler are applied to strategic areas such as nasal labial folds (deep folds on either side of the nose and mouth), at the hairline for a brow lift, and in droopy earlobes (from repeated wearing of heavy earrings) to tighten them. In the right hands, there's no bruising or downtime. Depending on the provider, costs begin at $600 for Restylane and Juvéderm, $800 for Sculptra.

Skin Tightening

This noninvasive procedure uses radio frequency with an FDA-approved machine known as the EndyMed 3Deep to firm and tighten skin and stimulate collagen. It represents an alternative in professional treatments for women of color. With skin tightening, it doesn't matter what color your skin is because the treatment addresses the multiple layers beneath the skin's surface. For those who love immediate gratification, skin tightening is a plus in that it offers both immediate and long-term benefits with repeated treatments. "You get an immediate tightening for a day or two, then the skin slowly tightens over time with repeated treatments," Dr. Ingleton says. If a patient is committed to the process, between three to six treatments are administered once a week or every two weeks until the desired results are achieved. Many women have it done above the brow to lift sagging eyelids (celebs have it done to open up their eyes prior to a big event); others have it done on the décolletage, under the chin, or on the neck as well as on the body to treat cellulite. During the procedure, a gel is applied to the skin and a treatment applicator is placed over the skin to obtain images of your skin to guide the treatment. A tingling sensation is experienced as the energy is delivered to the deeper layers of your skin. The process takes from an hour to an hour and a half and requires no downtime, though you may notice some temporary redness, swelling, or tenderness post treatment. Costs for skin tightening vary depending on the provider and the areas of treatment, with price ranges on average starting at $350 (brow) or $400 (jawline or neck).

Mesotherapy

This treatment originated in France, where injections of various medications were administered into the middle layer, or mesoderm, of the skin. Today, this FDA-approved treatment is used to improve skin tone, elasticity, and loss of facial volume. Also known as vitamin cocktails, the procedure incorporates vitamins to promote collagen and elastin and, if deemed appropriate by your professional, hyaluronic acid, resulting in plumper, firmer, hydrated skin that glows. NYC plastic surgeon Dr. Shirley Madhere administers VitaGlow microinjections (which originated in mesotherapy) of a combination of multivitamins and antioxidants, with or without hyaluronic acid, to complement surgical or nonsurgical techniques in facial rejuvenation and age management to skin of color. Vitamins that are typically injected include, but are not limited to, vitamins B, C, and E, as well as the elements selenium, copper, zinc, and manganese. The vitamin cocktail is absorbed into the skin, and the residual is "sealed" with a cooling facial mask. Madhere advises her patients to have a facial and a professional microdermabrasion treatment two to three days in advance to remove dead skin cells. If this isn't possible, a gentle facial scrub on the morning of the procedure will suffice. In preparation for this treatment, I exfoliated my skin as part of my morning cleansing. When I arrived at Madhere's fashionable downtown office, I was impressed by the thorough consultation that discussed the treatment in detail and, after an assessment, the ingredients that would be used to address my concerns: dryness and dull and uneven skin tone. In addition to vitamins B and E, extra C would be incorporated to address both dullness and pigmentary concerns along with hyaluronic acid to increase hydration and bring back my lost radiance. After my skin was cleansed, the injections were administered, and even though I needed a second round given that my winter-weary skin was so dry, I found them to be quick and painless. Once the injected vitamins were absorbed, Dr. Madhere applied a cooling, customized mask to suit my skin's needs, which to my pleasant surprise included turmeric, a natural anti-inflammatory. The entire procedure took place in approximately twenty minutes, and the results were immediate. My skin glowed like it does on a summer day! The next day I woke up with such an improved texture that I even did a double take! Results from the super skin nutrition, increased radiance and firmness, last up to one week after the first session and progressively increase in duration after at least three biweekly sessions due to the stimulation of collagen. Again, collagen, which declines with age, is one of the most abundant proteins in the body and is not only essential for the health and appearance of your skin, but also has everything to do with how you age, which in skin of color means fine lines and sagging. The results are enhanced by using skin care products at home that hydrate and also help to stimulate collagen. Side effects may include minor swelling or bruising, though I experienced neither. Costs range from $400 to $600 on average.

The road to great skin is paved by the right choices, not good intentions!

Mikki-ism

In a Class by Ourselves . . .

Here's what you need to know to manage pigmentary concerns, facial hair, and flesh moles.

Hyperpigmentation: On Your Mark

Managing hyperpigmentation (an overproduction of melanin)—which can be caused by sun damage, inflammation, birth control pills, hormonal influences, an injury, or even professional skin care treatments—can be a challenge as there's no rhyme or reason to the way melanin settles in our skin. It can be especially resistant on areas of repeated friction that the body perceives as an "injury," as on the elbows or the knees. Hyperpigmentation can also be symptomatic of certain illnesses such as autoimmune and gastrointestinal diseases or vitamin deficiencies, or as a side effect of certain medications such as antibiotics, chemotherapy, antiseizure drugs, and more.

In Office

Though hydroquinone (a skin-lightening ingredient) has been under scrutiny in previous years (with some evidence of carcinogenicity, though its potential in humans is unknown), dermatologists are still using this depigmenting agent. However, they are combining it with other proven ingredients, among them glycolic, kojic, and azelaic acids and retinoids, as part of an effective approach. Dr. Sumayah Taliaferro says the controversy surrounding hydroquinone, which continues to be investigated by the FDA, introduced new alternatives that dermatologists could use in treating pigmentary concerns: "I almost always use those ingredients [azelaic acid, kojic acid, licorice root] so we don't have to rely solely on hydroquinone for treatment." Antioxidants are also incorporated in treatment therapies. "Often when I treat a patient with melasma, I will not only recommend hydroquinone cream for the dark patches at night, I'll also recommend a vitamin C serum in the morning," Dr. Taliaferro says. "Vitamin C is a potent antioxidant, one that inhibits the enzyme tyrosinase, so it helps prevent melanin production," adds Dr. Cook-Bolden. Postinflammatory hyperpigmentation is a huge concern that requires fading the areas of spotty discoloration without incurring the halo or ghost effect caused by hydroquinone to the surrounding area, even from the most careful applications, and here again experts are calling on alternative ingredients to lighten and decrease inflammation. Alternative ingredients are also called upon in terms of skin tone to help "blend everything together," as Dr. Taliaferro puts it, to even the complexion without bleaching it. When hydroquinone is prescribed or found in professional lines like those available in office, it is available at pharmaceutical levels of 4 percent to effectively address resistant hyperpigmentation. Treatments like microdermabrasion, chemical peels, or laser therapy are also being incorporated to help speed results, but again, experts caution us—especially those of us with deeper skin tones—against having it done by dermatologists who aren't experienced with skin of color. "I have treated patients from other dermatologists where chemical peels have gone wrong," Taliaferro explains, "and that pigmentation is so significant that it takes years to improve that which occurred from a chemical peel when discoloration is the very thing they were trying to treat." But in the right hands, peels are an effective solution. Yours Truly had a glycolic peel to address my resistant dark elbows, and it made all the difference. But I must tell you, I should have kept up an at-home maintenance treatment since bending my elbows isn't optional!

At Home

Treating hyperpigmentation on your own, especially on your face, calls for applying fade products specifically to the pigmented area, and products like Ambi Fade Cream, which contains 2 percent hydroquinone and alpha hydroxy acid (fruit acid), and Nadinola Skin Discoloration Fade Cream, which contains 3 percent hydroquinone are recommended. There are alternative products that have emerged that make the application process more precise, like Sisley's Dark Spot Corrector, which has a roller-ball tip designed for targeted application and contains such active ingredients as stabilized vitamin C and salicylic acid. Dermatologists like NYC's Dr. Doris Day as well as Dr. Susan Evans recommend Oxygenetix Oxygenating Foundation Acne Control with SPF 25, which is available in a host of shades that work for the lightest to the deepest skin tones and contains several acne-fighting agents, time-released salicylic acid (2 percent), and Ceravitae, an oxygen complex that promotes collagen production. Another derm fave is Glytone Enhance Brightening Complex, which contains antioxidants to help brighten and protect the skin against future sun damage and 3 percent concentration of glycolic acid and 12 percent azelaic acid to gently exfoliate and inhibit the production of pigment. There's also Trufora Night Serum, which contains "bio-retinols" (vitamin A–free retinol alternatives), along with ingredients like vitamins C and E, organic aloe vera, and oat extract. "I love this product for my sensitive and vegan patients," notes Dr. Cook-Bolden.

Facial Hair

Excessive facial hair among women of color is often caused by hormonal changes and can be coarse, thick, and more noticeable. Deeper skin tones are susceptible to trauma during removal that can result in discoloration, burning, scarring, and pseudofolliculitis barbae, where curly, coarse hairs pierce and reenter the skin causing inflammation and razor bumps.

In Office

Removal is influenced by the amount of hair, and today laser therapy (where energy is sent through the follicle to destroy the root) is the treatment of choice. Here again I advise you to make sure to see a board-certified dermatologist who's experienced with skin of color. Thanks to technology, now even those of us with deep skin tones can safely take this route without concern due to the Nd:YAG laser, as it doesn't affect the skin's color but effectively removes dark facial hair with no downtime. According to Dr. Taliaferro, successful treatment has a lot to do with how you treat your skin beforehand. "It's extremely important not to use exfoliators or cleansers that contain glycolic acid or salicylic acid. Doing so will cause adverse effects," she warns. Though not entirely painless, several laser treatments result in permanent hair removal. Combination therapy is also part of the plan of action that sees many dermatologists incorporating microdermabrasion or chemical peels in treating skin of color so it stays in the clear. We can also benefit from electrolysis, where a fine probe/needle administers an electrical spark to the pore to burn out the follicle and prevent regrowth.

Alternatives

Threading, a process where the hair is entwined in the thread and lifted out of the follicle, is another option if hair growth is minimal. Waxing at salons and spas, though temporary, represents a quick option; however, choosing a reputable location is key because skin infections are possible.

At Home

Waxing kits and depilatories recommended for the face can efficiently remove hair; however, you should do a patch test first to check for any possible reactions. With waxing, there is the possibility of discoloration as it does present a form of trauma to the skin with the repeated pulling out of hair. Depilatories don't always work efficiently on coarse hair, and if you have sensitive skin or leave them on too long, you can risk irritation or chemical burns from the active ingredient of calcium thioglycolate and/or potassium thioglycolate. Vaniqa is also useful; however, it only slows down hair growth.

Flesh Moles

Otherwise known as dermatosis papulosa nigra, these hereditary skin growths made up of cells that range from dark brown to black in color can occur all over the face and upper body area singularly or in small clusters increasingly with age.

In Office

If you choose to remove flesh moles, laser treatment offers the most minimal side effects. The Nd:YAG laser is the safest choice for dark skin tones. Flesh moles are also removed through a process known as electrodessication, where they are burned or seared with an electric current that passes through a wire, causing them to fall off without scarring. There is, however, a temporary risk of discoloration that eventually fades. Though flesh moles can also be frozen using liquid nitrogen, where super cold liquid nitrogen is applied and the mole is allowed to fall off, derms like Dr. Taliaferro caution against this procedure as liquid nitrogen can cause one to develop hypopigmentation (loss of melanin).

Shop Talk: Maximizing Your MVPs

A skin of color glossary to put you in the know about the A-plus ingredients that perform for us:

- **Hyaluronic acid:** Renowned for its ability to retain moisture (holds up to a thousand times its weight in water); plumps and repairs, imparts radiance, smooths fine lines; used in topical skin care like serums and moisturizers; used in fillers to plump and firm for its compatibility with the human body.
- **Salicylic acid:** An "active" ingredient that clears breakouts and prevents them from reoccurring, treats whiteheads and blackheads; anti-inflammatory, antimicrobial; has exfoliating properties; great at clearing pores of sebum and dirt; used in topical skin care as well as in chemical peels.
- **Licorice extract:** Anti-inflammatory, skin-soothing; an effective melanin inhibitor; used in topical skin care.
- **Niacinamide:** Improves microcirculation, stimulates collagen, enhances elasticity, inhibits hyperpigmentation; anti-inflammatory; used in topical skin care.
- **Arbutin:** A natural skin lightener; works by blocking the formation of melanin, which is activated by UV light; used in topical skin care and professional treatments.
- **Azeleic acid:** Treats acne; used in topical skin care products.
- **Bearberry extract:** Natural skin lightener (often combined with other ingredients to avoid overbleaching); fights free radicals; used in topical skin care products.
- **Peptides:** Proteins that stimulate collagen; replenishes, firms, improves fine lines; used in topical skin care products.
- **Retinol:** Vitamin A derivative, gold standard ingredient for speeding cell turnover, promoting firmness, diminishing fine lines, resurfacing skin texture, reducing hyperpigmentation; used in topical skin care products and professional treatments.

- **Glycolic acid:** Exfoliates, regenerates collagen, breaks up pigment cells; used in topical skin care as well as professional treatments.
- **Vitamin C:** Brightening, disrupts melanin; top age-defying antioxidant, stimulates cells to make collagen; used in topical skin care products as well as professional treatments.
- **Green tea:** Antioxidant; protects from sun damage; inhibits collagen and elastin breakdown, reduces excess sebum and inflammation; used in topical skin care products.
- **Squalane:** Derived from sugar cane; replenishes intrinsic hydration, increases cell turnover; great catalyst for other ingredients; used in topical skin care products.
- **Ferulic acid:** Antioxidant, anti-inflammatory; diminishes hyper-pigmentation.

Aging Fabulous

As a beauty girl, I'll be the first to tell you that technology should be calling you and you should be having a great time examining your options and discovering your best skin ever. The truth about us and aging is that we wear it *youthfully well*, but that doesn't mean we don't experience our own unique effects. We get that the stressors of modern-day life, changing environmental concerns, and the challenges that come with time call for us to be proactive and in the know no matter what birthday is on the horizon, and we're showing up ready. We sisters love being ahead of the game, and when it comes to our beautiful brown skin, we're on it. Here's a primer for the ages:

Twenties

Commonalities
Acne, oiliness, premenstrual breakouts, postinflammatory pigmentation.

Pro Take

Even though skin during this decade is plump and in a state of optimal renewal, now is a time for consistent prevention and a good regimen. "So it's cleanse, put your antioxidants (vitamins A, C, E) on your skin and your sunscreen. We don't even talk astringent anymore as it's just taking oils away," Dr. Ingleton advises. If breakouts or acne is a concern, don't pick or self-treat. It's important to consult the experts to prevent exacerbation or postinflammatory pigmentation and keep your skin in the clear. At this stage, many derms recommend topical treatments to control breakouts and, for acne, a cocktail of ingredients and treatments depending on the severity. "We treat acne with vitamin A, salicylic acid, 2 percent bearberry for lightening and to decrease inflammation," says Dr. Evans. Retinols, glycolic acid, and lactic acid are also called into play by the pros to stimulate collagen and keep skin smooth and glowing. Know, too, that everything from yo-yo dieting to birth control pills have an effect on the skin. The former causes it to lose elasticity, while the latter, even though it may clear up acne, has been associated with melasma. So, again, using a broad-spectrum sunscreen and an appropriate fade solution may also be advised.

Thirties

Commonalities

Fine expression lines, discoloration, texture changes, facial hair, "adult acne."

Pro Take

Minimal signs of aging can appear, like those fine lines you now notice under the eyes from repeated expressions or frowning. Hyperpigmentation concerns may surface (see "Hyperpigmentation: On Your Mark," page 105) and may require you to seek professional treatment, depending on its cause, to choose the mildest options to check it. Texture changes due to slowed cell renewal may show up. Just let it remind you to step up your care game with nutritious ingredients that address your need for hydration and keep you in the glow. Here an aesthetician or dermatologist may recommend adding a serum like vitamin C to your regimen, or monthly facials and perhaps microdermabrasion or a mild peel to help retexturize the skin and stimulate collagen. Aside from these factors, acne may show up for the first time and call for a treatment approach that will address it without drying out your skin.

Forties

Commonalities
Dryness, sagging, frown lines, lack of radiance, facial hair.

Pro Take
You've taken on the world and are having your say, but now's the time to show a little more love to the woman in the mirror. Skin may have become drier and a little less radiant, and declining levels of estrogen, which maintain collagen and elastin, *may* begin to show up as a lack of firmness. There may also be a few frown lines in your selfie! Early menopause may cause an increase in facial hair. Existing skin care products may need to shift as they may no longer meet your needs and desires. If you haven't begun to partner with an aesthetician and a dermatologist, you certainly want to consider doing so now. Many ingredients listed in the skin care glossary (see "Shop Talk: Maximizing Your MVPs," page 110) can help promote collagen production and increase hydration as well as the radiance you desire—both at the hands of your skin care professional as well as in the many dermatological product picks. If the deepening "parenthesis" (nasal labial folds) concern you, or if anywhere the plumpness you're accustomed to has begun to slacken or seemingly decline, fillers can be used to subtly tweak these areas to your joy. Frown lines and crow's-feet can be dramatically softened with Botox. Facial

hair, which can cause complications for women of color, may need to be addressed, whether at home or by a dermatologist.

Fifties and Beyond

Commonalities

Crow's-feet, unevenness, dryness, deeper lines around the nose and mouth, sagging.

Pro Take

The onset of menopause can bring about a slowed production of estrogen and less collagen production, which may show up more pronounced on some than others. I remember my mother still had her plump cheeks and ultrasmooth skin that glowed at age sixty-seven, so the old adage "It's in the genes" still holds true among us, which is why a lot of times it's not your chronological age but the age of your skin that matters. Nevertheless, this is the time when experts commonly see a slight loss of firmness among us "grown girls," as Ledisi would say, along with crow's-feet and fine lines under the eyes. Sebaceous glands secrete less oil, and so skin is usually drier and can appear lackluster. A nurturing regimen of antioxidants as well as those that specifically address texture, tone, and firmness is important. Crow's-feet and fine lines can be softened with an eye cream that contains peptides or retinol. For Yours Truly, a regimen that includes hyaluronic acid, vitamin C, and peptides is a click for the way I like my overall skin to look. Everyone knows I'm a smiler, so it finally caught up with me at age sixty-three, when the expression folds around my nose, mouth, and eyes seemingly came to stay, and since I live in "test-girl mode," I decided to give injectables a try. In the conservative hands of Dr. Cook-Bolden, I had Restylane to slightly fill the area on either side of my nose as well as less than a syringe of Botox to smooth the line between my brows and the "sparrow feet," as I call them, around my eyes. (They haven't grown into crow's-feet yet!) And I like the results. Did I have any trepidation? Of course, for about five minutes! I was quite comfortable after the very thorough consultation and the thought that I was taking a power step, as I have throughout my reporting career, because I could then tell you firsthand about the experience. I've never been one of those gals who tell others, "Do as I say, not as I do!" For me, Botox lasted surprisingly well and didn't begin to subside until five months after treatment, while the filler's decline wasn't visible until six months later. There was no downtime. In fact, I taped a show the next day. Enough said.

You Better Work!
Strategies, Solutions, and Time-Honored Picks

Instant Gratification

Every Queen needs a pick-me-up when she's short on rest and big on Instagram! Here are my recovery faves for hitting the scene photo-ready: SK-II Facial Treatment Masks (fab sheets that renew the skin), Nars Laguna Illuminator (a light-reflecting liquid that enhances chocolate skin with a golden shimmer), baby oil and sea salt (a quick DIY body exfoliator), and Johnson & Johnson Baby Oil Gel for a gleam finish. When time is on my side, wonderful therapeutic hydration masks (they're gel-filled and reusable) increase the hydration in your skin by 180 percent, leaving it ultra-fresh. I slip one on for forty minutes before going out, and voilà, a fresh finish is on!

Revival Time

Post holiday, post winter, post illness, restoring your skin calls for a strategy. How to? Begin with a purifying cleanser to restore clarity and remove dead cells without stripping to detoxify your skin and improve your texture. Follow this with a clarifying clay mask if you have oily skin, an enzyme mask if you have combination skin, or a hydrating mask to nourish dry skin via the supercharged ingredients they now deliver. I've also found those that are meant to be slept in and some that work their magic in less than ten minutes, leaving your skin as smooth as a baby's bottom. Follow with a radiance-boosting serum, and then seal the deal with a moisturizer with SPF. In fact, next time you have the gals over, why not have a mask-querade party? It's a fun way to fellowship. Here's looking at you!

Back in Action

For those searing days, or hot-ticket nights when you want to pop on a dress with a little exit-ness, make sure you've got back—as in one that's smooth and in the clear. Listen, skin is skin, and the same flare-ups and challenges that can occur on the face can pop up on your back at any time. Given what a style setter you are, the last thing you'll want to have cramp your look are such concerns as back acne (backne), hyperpigmentation, clogged pores, or poor texture. Don't sweat it. Consider having a back facial. Much like a standard facial, the basic process involves cleansing, exfoliation, extractions, and a mask. Options also include glycolic peels and microdermabrasion. At home, use an antibacterial facial cleanser to check breakouts and keep pores in the clear. If your skin is on the dry side, consider a light, noncomedogenic body lotion with soothing oatmeal like Aveeno Daily Moisturizing Lotion. Now, who's got your back?

Sparse Brows

Brows are the frame of the face, and for those who have sparse brows or brows in "absentee," like mine, microblading, also referred to as 3-D embroidery or a "feathered brow," is a very natural option. Whether you've experienced a poor waxing job, overplucked, undergone chemotherapy and are two years out from their treatments, or have trichotillomania, alopecia, or a disorder that has led to hair loss, this process is a game changer. It's also great for those with oily skin for whom pencils don't hold up well. Microblading is the technique of implanting pigment under your skin using a microblade to simulate hair strokes and create fuller-looking brows. Unlike tattoo artists, who use ink whose finish is like a solid block of color and can look harsh, microblading artists use pigment. "With microblading, because it's just deposited under the top layer of the skin, looks like hair, and because it's semiperma-nent (it fades out in twelve to eighteen months), you're not stuck so you can change your style," says NYC brow artist Patricia Cameron, who's known for re-creating existing brows—or, if a client has none, a "neighbor," as she calls it at her Beauty and the Brow salon in Midtown. During consultation, your cus-tom brow shape, based on your bone structure and your desires, along with your best hue, is determined. Once your shape and best pigment are set, the skin is primed—or shall I say prickled (it feels like fine needles across the brow area)—with a skin-numbing liquid lidocaine, and the one- to two-hour pro-cess of creating hairlike strokes begins. Results are astonishingly natural, a big time-saver to your morning makeup routine, and cost-effective as you need nothing—no more brow pencils, powder, etc.—to maintain perfect brows. And follow-up care after the procedure is simple but essential to their longevity. Cameron cautions, "You can't get them wet for at least a week. That means using a shower cap to cover them, no washing your face with water because, until they actually heal, water will flush out the effect." That also meant no sweaty workouts for Ms. Mikki! After the procedure is done, brows may appear darker during the healing phase but will fade after you begin to wash your face again. Any scabbing that may occur while you heal tends to look like more hair (really nice for a gal like me!) Following your initial session, there is a touch-up appointment after four to eight weeks to discuss any desired tweaks. This is where artists like Cameron add more color, strokes, or definition depending on client preferences. Who's not a candidate for microblading? Women who are taking blood thinners, have had Botox two weeks prior, or have a history of keloid scarring or severe acne. Costs for the initial procedure range from $600 to $900, depending on the provider. In terms of downtime, it depends on the person. Though most go about life as usual, it's best for first-timers to prepare for a week of no commitments. "A lot of my clients go back to work, they go to social events, and they go on dates where they get compliments during the healing phase," says Cameron, who finds the adjustment during the initial phase is more about getting used to having more pronounced brows. I'm hap-py to say I continued with my nonstop schedule as usual.

Under-Eye Bags

Under-eye bags can be caused by fluid retention, lack of sleep, allergies, and more; however, the real issue that commands one's attention is when they come to stay via the aging process. There are effective topical products like serums, gels, and cooling roll-ons that contain caffeine, which instantly reduces swelling. A more permanent offering lies in fillers. "Great for those who don't want surgery and have just a little bit of volume under the eye," says Madhere. An injectable of Restylane, the popular hyaluronic acid filler, or a syringe of one's own body fat are both widely used by doctors to address this concern. Injectables in this area last approximately six months and may require you to plan for some downtime for bruising and swelling. Costs range from approximately $650 to $950 per syringe. So it really comes down to deciding whether you're looking for a temporary or a long-term solution. In the meantime, don't sleep on your face, as this will encourage fluids to collect under your eyes. Instead, sleep on your back, and on late nights, do add an extra pillow. In this case, you'll want to apply a serum before bed that calms inflammation and boosts collagen: try This Works No Wrinkles Tired Eyes stimulating serum, which is designed to work while you sleep. Again, don't sleep in makeup as it can irritate your eyes and cause puffiness as well. Finally, know that what you toast with and how many glasses of spirits you have will also turn up in the morning as puffiness.

Extended Play

Enviable legs call for a velvety smoothness that's visible to the naked eye. Come spring, if you're like most dolls who live in a seasonal climate and like to drop the hose and work flirtatious hemlines with knockout heels, then a bit of prep is in order. Your first order of business is to satinize your skin with an exfoliant. I like a two-pronged approach for my reveal, so I exfoliate weekly with a salt scrub and a loofah, coupled with the daily use of a chemical exfoliant, such as an alpha hydroxy or glycolic acid lotion to speed up the shedding of dead skin cells. If you have to defuzz, waxing, Revitol or Kalo (both are hair-growth inhibitors that are available online), or lasers (make sure to see a board-certified dermatologist who's experienced with skin of color) all represent solutions. Begin to work on any discoloration well in advance with an over-the-counter product containing hydroquinone and, if resistant, schedule a consultation with a dermatologist for such options as a prescription-strength fade formula that might combine hydroquinone with retinoids to improve penetration and glycolic acid to break up stubborn pigment. He or she might also integrate microdermabrasion or a chemical peel for better results. Once you've achieved your desired effect, get ready to "glow for it" by incorporating the use of a tinted self-tanner or schedule a professional spray-tanning session as sallow legs aren't an option!

Master Class

- Banish spider or varicose veins during the winter months (while you're still in hose or can rely on slacks for cover) by seeing a vascular specialist for sclerotherapy (for the former) or endovenous laser ablation (for the latter).
- Tone up and show out with consistent cardio and strength training such as squats, lunges, calf raises, bar work, leg lifts, and taking the stairs whenever possible, two at a time.
- Gleam up when your beauty mission is accomplished with a light body oil and sizzle day in and day out!

It's the Small Things That Count

When it comes to beauty, I'll take maintenance and treatment over correction anyday. It's always better to stay on top things than to fall behind. Good beauty habits are what keep your look intact and life simple. What's also important is having a stash of products that can come to the rescue in a "beauty emergency." Here's what should be in your medicine cabinet:

- Got that zit that popped up out of nowhere? Mario Badescu Drying Lotion, a spot treatment that shrinks zits and whiteheads overnight.

- Scorched yourself while cooking? Kelo-cote Advanced Formula Scar Gel to minimize inflammation and speed healing.
- Skinned yourself? iS Clinical Sheald Recovery Balm to begin repairing skin immediately; ScarAway Silicone Scar Sheets, which offers the same silicone technology used by plastic surgeons, to prevent scarring—it's also an effective treatment for scars new or old.
- Woke up with red, puffy eyes? Bausch + Lomb Opcon-A eye drops to clear redness, reduce itching, and Clinique All About Eyes Serum, a roll-on, to cool and de-puff, and a doc-in-a box eye cream like Estée Lauder's Re-Nutriv Ultimate Diamond Transformative Energy Eye Creme.
- Unsightly cold sore? Abreva cold sore treatment, a prescription-strength formula that speeds healing on contact.

My Must-Haves

Someone once asked me what was the one thing I couldn't live without on a desert island. My response: "Spare me, I wouldn't go! I don't have one thing I can't live without!" Here are my beauty must-haves:

1 My Bible
2 Multipurpose cleanser
3 De-puffing eye cream
4 Moisturizer with SPF 30
5 Argan oil
6 Lip balm
7 Shea butter
8 Vitamins
9 Paddle brush
10 Silk head wrap

Notes to Self...

Notes to Self...

3

Makeup: No Limits!

On most days, my office looks like "Beauty UPS," meaning there are products everywhere, and as a result, I stay in "test mode." For sure there are those picks that make me say "Yassss!" and then there are those that make me say, "Well, that's a toss!" Like you, I'm always on the lookout for new finds even beyond the many press and product deliveries that I get for review. I'm the one who's always asking makeup artists what's in their stash. I hit beauty destinations everywhere I go, from the best drugstores (yes, I'm a drugstore gal who loves a great find) across the country to duty-free exclusives and all the best-kept secret spots of the pros (like Alcone and Inglot in New York and "the Alley" in LA) and beauty shows where those in the know get the new and the next. I've even gone to Cosmoprof in Bologna, Italy, the international hub where vast numbers of exhibitors and decision makers meet to showcase and decide the future in beauty. For someone like Yours Truly, it's the "Land of Oz" in beauty. There's a whole new world out there compared to what it used to be, where foundations masked our skin and the natural nuances that we love or where beauty companies offered women of color a limited range of textures. But nowadays more of us are color chemists and decision makers at beauty companies, and we ourselves, as beauty buyers, have become more vocal, so the makeup that appeals now is predicated on visionary "second skin" formulas, textures, and hues, so when coupled with surefire techniques, we can go from fresh and fearless to fierce and fabulous with ease!

No one wants to work hard for a look, nor should they. After all, who has the time? This is the future we dreamed of, and only performance-driven picks that work fast and fabulous with lasting results are worthy of a purchase. In reality, everything in your life should earn its space and help you *slay*, especially that which plays the distinctive role in how you express your beauty. Though products abound and great finds can be had at every price point, be selective, choose with your desires and, again, your lifestyle in mind, and before you buy anything, decide how you want to express yourself, be it a look that's utterly fresh, one that's totally glam, or as bold and authentic as you wanna be!

66 **M**any people think beauty is determined by the outcome, but self-appreciation goes just as far!"

—Reggie Wells, celebrity makeup artist

Don't let anything get in the way of expressing your beauty. Think of it as your "noncompete clause" for life!

Mikki-ism

Be Clear

A great look hinges on taking impeccable care of your skin and setting time for grooming practices (e.g., removing facial hair and shaping your brows) that impact the results you want, especially if you're a gal who subscribes to a "less is more" look. There's nothing wrong with being "high maintenance" when it comes your beauty, and I say spare no expense when it comes to taking care of your skin and putting your best face forward. The way I see it, membership has its privileges, and you're not only worth it, but it's a great time-saver in your day-to-day.

> 66 **T**rends come and go, but a perfect brow everyone wants."
>
> —Sam Fine, celebrity makeup artist

Let's Browse

A polished look always rests on how well one's brows are defined. Most brow experts favor a look that's clean, well tapered, and slightly filled in. To achieve your best look, consult a pro, as this takes away the guesswork, and once your best brows are in place, you can work it from there. Here's what you need to know to stay in shape:

- ◉ Choose a hair-removal method that you can keep up. If your hair is fine and you need minimal shaping to maintain it, a good slanted tweezer and a magnifying mirror are your best bets. If your brows are thick and coarse, this is where I recommend professional waxing in the hands of a true pro so it's precise, quick, and painless!

◉ If your brow hairs are long, brush them up and trim those that extend beyond your basic brow line. Comb hairs down and repeat. Then, brush them back into your basic shape and tweeze any stray hairs that fall beneath the brow bone. You should only grip individual hairs when tweezing. Never grab clusters in an effort to get it done faster or you'll be left with gaping holes (not pretty), and make sure to remove hairs in the direction in which they grow.

◉ To shape, fill in any sparse areas using a brow pencil and complete the look using a slanted brow brush and brow powder as layering will give you the most natural finish. The basics call for you to use a shade that closely matches your brow color. Never go darker in hue as it's hard, aging, and tends to look drawn on and fake—in short, it will give you the kind of look that makes an entrance before you do. Very unflattering. If that's not enough, it will weigh your look down. Makeup artists like Ashunta Sheriff, who keeps Taraji P. Henson's look in demand, take it a step further by reminding us that brows aren't uniform in color and look most natural when that is taken into consideration. "I'm an avid believer of bringing some highlight to brows with this in mind," Ashunta says. This step creates dimension and keeps brows from looking too done. Renee Garnes, whose clients include Naomi Campbell, Zoë Kravitz, and Alfre Woodard, says it's about paying attention to the seemingly small details: "I always match brow color to the root of the hair, so it's not so color-by-number, and then I brush the brow so the finish is soft and natural and not so drawn that it looks like Etch A Sketch."

◉ If your brows are absentee, try this approach: Tap a matte primer, like Becca Ever-Matte Poreless Priming Perfector, on your brow bone to check oil, create a matte surface, and hold your brow products in place. Next, use a brow stencil, as they take the guesswork out of the application as you simply lay the stencil on your brow bone and fill it in using a brow powder as the basis for your best brow. Remove the stencil and then fill in with a brow pencil. I recommend doing so with a good moisture-resistant brow pencil like MAC Cosmetics Eye Brows so they'll hold fast. You could also consider having microblading (see "Sparse Brows," page 116), a process that implants pigment under your skin using a microblade to simulate hair strokes and create fuller-looking brows. As a more permanent option, you can also have an eyebrow transplant.

Looking "done" is over and out. Now creatively injecting personality into a look, that's another thing entirely.

Mikki-ism

Tool It Up!

Brush with Greatness

You can spend or be thrifty when it comes to makeup buys, but do be partial to a good set of quality makeup brushes that will be kind to your skin, retain their shape, and cleanse easily. You can purchase a pre-packaged set from any of the top cosmetic counters, or you can make individual picks at destination spots like Sephora, MAC, Ulta, or Bobbi Brown. As for maintenance, always store your brushes in a case. Cleanse them weekly with a makeup brush cleanser or baby shampoo, as oil and bacteria can build up on the bristles. Always rinse well, squeeze, and allow them to dry flat on a rack (like a small inexpensive cake rack). In a pinch, you can also use a brush spray until you have time to shampoo them. Now, here are your MVPs:

- **Foundation brush:** The pilot for even coverage and a seamless application.

- **Concealer brush:** Perfect cover-up tool for blending and application under eyes and around the nose.

- **Blush brush:** For sweeping powder blush on accurately, minus the telltale edges.

- **Powder brush:** The perfect duster for face powder or bronzer.

- **Flat shadow brush:** For precise application of color on lids.

- **Fluffy medium-size shadow brush:** Great for building color.

- **Blending brush:** Makes blending/softening shadow in the crease effortless.

- **Angled liner brush:** For precision eye lining.

- **Slanted brow brush:** For filling in brows.

- **Eyebrow spoolie:** For smoothing and unifying brows and softening excess product.

- **Lip brush:** For precise application of color, coverage, and merging lip picks and liner.

Beauty Box: Well Blended

Today's makeup sponges give new meaning to defining a flawless canvas and are a pick that every gal should have. Hands down, makeup artist Rea Ann Silva, who I first met on a cover shoot with actress Sheryl Lee Ralph, changed the game when it came to sponges in creating the BeautyBlender. It's a must-have among editors and makeup artists alike that Rea developed while she was working on the hit TV show *Girlfriends* with Tracee Ellis Ross to perfect the art of creating a flawless look and maintaining it through touch-ups in the face of high-def cameras. What I love about this now classic pick is its multitasking ability to apply foundation seamlessly, touch up on the go, *and* wipe out shine without disturbing your makeup. It's also a perfect pick for women of a certain age to check perspiration when inner temps rise, as it can get soaked and still not absorb your foundation. For Ashunta, who uses the "genius tool," as she calls it, on Taraji, the trick is in the buffing as it makes the skin look fresh and healthy. Before the BeautyBlender, sponges were a disposable item, most often purchased by the bag, used once, and tossed. With the arrival of the BeautyBlender in its happiness-inducing hot-pink hue, taking advantage of new technology that makes it gentle, washable, and reusable, came a plethora of industry knockoffs in various shapes that allow you to control foundation and concealer coverage, contour, blend, blush, and apply powder, all with a seamless finish. Sponges like these require a little more maintenance, but they're worth it as they can last up to two months (maybe more if you're not a big makeup wearer) if you clean them with a cleanser specified for this purpose after each use and store them in a ventilated container. You never want to store them in a ziplock bag while damp as the moisture will cause bacteria to grow which can invite breakouts. At $20 the BeautyBlender is an investment pick and the leader of the pack; however, you can purchase bargain buys starting at $5 at beauty destinations like Ulta, and Ricky's NYC.

---

66 I really pride myself on making the skin look natural and not so made up. Even though you're painted, you're not painted to the gods."

—Renee Garnes, celebrity makeup artist

AFFIRMATION

It's not how beautiful your makeup is; it's how beautiful *you* are. That can't be purchased!

Next of Skin

Think of today's base products, those all-important picks like primer, base, concealer, and powder, as you do underpinnings, and look to them to support, smooth, perfect, and, where necessary, camouflage. Your look is the star here, everything else is the backdrop, which is why layering is more important now than ever. I remember visiting John Legend in the studio for a "listening session" one evening for his new music, and while there I learned how music tracks are layered to achieve a seamless sound. Foundational products are a lot like that inasmuch as their purpose is to achieve a seamless look. Here it's about making the right choices and identifying what your desires are on this basic level.

66 The key about makeup now is looking like you were born with this skin."

—Toni Acey, celebrity makeup artist

Blurred Lines

Face primers are like the Facetune app in beauty as they, too, smooth your skin and convincingly blur your pores, whether you wear foundation or not. If you do wear base, face primers give your foundation the kind of longevity that causes it to keep your pace from morning till night. Makeup artist Toni Acey says, "Like any great painting, you have to start with a smooth canvas as that will always ensure that your makeup is going to be as flawless as possible, even if your skin is a little textured." There are all kinds of formulations, from those that act as a mattifier, check oil, stop creasing, and target acne, to those that hydrate and impart radiance to dry or lackluster complexions. There are also primers for eyes and lips that lock color and product in place until you're ready to take it off. Think of it this way: when your days extend well beyond the nine-to-five, it's all about starting off with the right finish to avoid toting too many products in your makeup bag and to save time on touch-ups. Here's what will give you the edge that lasts:

Primer 101

⊚ **Face primer:** If you wear foundation, you want it to last and that's where a primer comes in. A primer is to foundation what a base coat is to nail polish: you shouldn't use one without the other. Primers not only allow your makeup to go on easily and stay put, but also make your skin appear ultrasmooth. They can be applied with a large sponge or by hand after your moisturizer.

⊙ **Eye shadow primer:** Everyone gets a little oily in the crease area, and that causes smudging. When you couple that with such culprits as humidity or even annoying allergies, then you know that such meltdowns aren't pretty! Makeup artist Sam Fine, who's behind the look of actress Queen Latifah, uses this analogy: "Think of primer as the antiperspirant for your face (in this case your eyes) and know that it's great to dry the surface, make the skin less porous and easier for product to adhere." This is when you can thank the beauty industry for coming to your rescue with the picks that protect your investment.

⊙ **Lip primer:** No matter how long-wearing your lipstick, a primer allows it to give you the most bang for your buck. It also perfects the surface of your lips, especially if you're a matte lipstick wearer because matte lipstick without a primer is never pretty.

Shopping Cart

- Becca Ever-Matte Poreless Priming Perfector
- Jay Manuel Beauty Face Tuning Primer
- Laura Mercier Foundation Primer—Oil Free
- Neutrogena Shine Control Primer
- bareMinerals Blemish Remedy Mattifying Prep Gel
- Smashbox 24 Hour Photo Finish Shadow Primer
- bareMinerals Prime Time Eyelid Primer
- MAC Prep + Prime Lip

Where coverage is concerned, one should think more "hide-and-chic" than simply "hide." You don't want to hide behind a wall of makeup!

Mikki-ism

What's your foundation objective? Color? Coverage? Complexion perfection? No matter your desires, the key lies in selecting the right formulation because, as in skin care, one size does not fit all. Lifestyle is also important, and I couldn't agree more with Fine, who believes the key to success lies in finding your makeup personality and catering to it. "A lot of women go to results first as opposed to their personality, what resonates with them, and how much time they have to dedicate to their beauty," Fine explains, "but just like the old adage 'Don't go shopping hungry, you'll buy everything,' the same holds true with foundation." There are so many taglines and marketing strategies that women are buying into and not realizing what's a fit and what's not. So hands down, you've got to think about what you'd be comfortable with before you shop. There are some guidelines that can help narrow your search. For example, if your skin is dry, you might want to think twice about a matte foundation, which can cause fine lines to be more prominent; however, if you're normal to oily, say "Hello!" Moisturizing or "satin" foundations are best for dry skin, and today's formulas look luminous, not greasy. Acey recommends going a step further by making sure the base products you choose don't undermine one another: "I like to make sure my foundation and my concealer are compatible. For example, if one is oil-based and the other is water-based, they're going to compete with one another." In other words, Acey maintains that if you use a water-based concealer, you should use a water-based foundation.

When shopping for your best base, always aim for a finish that's "weightless," "seamless," "fresh," and "unmasked," and give equal thought to the tool and the lighting in your home that will help you best achieve it. I have a vanity that I placed right in front of a window so I'm always guaranteed a flood of natural light because I don't want to be deceived when creating a look. When I didn't have the luxury of a vanity, I put a chair in front of the window and a good mirror. Because lighting is so important, it's about finding your best spot, whether it's the dining room table or "turning the kitchen island into your beauty area," as Fine says. Lighting aside, the great thing now is that you can achieve this look of "skinspiration," as some pros call it, at any price point. Acey, who serves as head makeup artist for the nationally televised special *Black Girls Rock!*, says, "You don't have to spend forty or fifty dollars now as a ten dollar foundation works just as well." The busy makeup artist, who can often be found on set in her home base of Atlanta due to the large influx of TV shows being produced there, notes that when HDTV arrived, HD products arrived, and technology is continuing to evolve, so base products are more refined and not so heavy. They also allow for more flexibility, so you can go from light to full coverage.

Still, the best foundation is only as good as its ability to match your skin. When it comes to color, makeup artists like Ashunta still favor the "jawline trick" of applying three stripes on your lower jawline to gauge your hue: "Choose three shades: one you know works, one you think works, and one that you know doesn't work; put the one that doesn't work in the middle and the one you think might work on one side and the one you know works on the other side, and whichever one just melts into your skin so close that you don't even see it, that's your shade." Since our hues seem to come and go at retail, I suggest that whenever you can find the same shade in different textures—liquid, stick, cream—make that move!

Base Strokes: Foundation Picks Now

- BB cream: Minimal coverage with skin care benefits.

- Liquid: Offers sheer to medium coverage; available in both matte and satin finishes.

- Cream: Provides medium to maximum coverage; available in oil-free and moisturizing formulas.

- Cream-to-powder: Offers medium to full coverage; matte, powder finish; suitable for all skin types.

- Stick: Provides medium to full coverage; semimatte finish; suitable for all skin types.

- Cream cushion: Sheer coverage; skin care benefits with an antibacterial sponge.

Shopping Cart

Product preferences vary for keeping your canvas fresh and flawless. Here are some great options:
- MAC Cosmetics Matchmaster SPF 15 Foundation
- Nars All Day Luminous Weightless Foundation
- Bobbi Brown Skin Weightless Powder Foundation
- Lancôme Miracle Cushion Liquid Cushion Compact Foundation

- CoverGirl Queen Collection Natural Hue Compact Foundation
- Clinique Even Better Glow Light Reflecting Makeup Broad Spectrum SPF 15
- Glamazon Beauty Second Skin Liquid Foundation
- Hourglass Vanish Seamless Finish Foundation Stick

Concealing the Matter

66 **A** good concealer works like a correction fluid works on paper. If you use the same color as your foundation, you're really not correcting the problem."

—Toni Acey, celebrity makeup artist

I'll be the first to say it: We all have a little something to hide, right? For Yours Truly, it's discoloration around my mouth from years of using whitening toothpaste. Who knew! For you it might be dark circles or dark spots. This is where concealer becomes your best beauty staple. Depending on your needs, shade and texture are everything. "All women of color need something that has a golden/peachy undertone because if we go with just a yellow undertone, it'll appear ashy," Ashunta says. It's important to go two or three shades lighter than your foundation, and though it might be tempting to use your foundation to conceal trouble spots, a lot of artists recommend getting a concealer instead. "Foundation is meant to even out skin tone, and concealers are meant to hide imperfections," Ashunta explains. Depending on the base you choose and the area where you need coverage, foundation might not hold up as well. Finding your texture fave is also essential, as some formulas are easier to work with than others and you need to know the difference. "I always try to find something that's moisturizing, not too dry, and not too wet, so it doesn't slide—then you'll get the coverage and the ease you need," says Garnes.

Beauty Box: Concealer

Whether you use concealer to hide undereye circles, or camouflage splotchiness or stubborn pigmentation, there's a multitasking formula that'll help you get even. Here's a list of formulations to help you decide your best consistency.

- **Cream:** Delivers full coverage.
- **Stick:** Provides medium coverage.
- **Liquid:** Affords light to medium coverage.
- **Wand:** Offers light, creamy coverage.

Shopping Cart

- MAC Pro Longwear Concealer (fluid): Medium to full matte coverage.
- Kat Von D Lock-It Concealer Crème (brush-on cream): Full coverage, waterproof, brightens dark circles.
- Bobbi Brown Creamy Concealer (cream): Maximum coverage.
- Black Opal True Color Flawless Perfecting Concealer (stick): Medium to full coverage.

Powder-ful

Powder often gets a bad rap, but when used properly, it can be a stroke of genius. Technology has driven out the old masking powders (but didn't kill the big red sponge a lot of gals used to use!), and whether you choose a pressed or loose version in your perfect shade, powder is a great way to not only set a finish and check unwanted shine but also look fresh and flawless. It's all in how you apply it. For example, you might choose to set your makeup in the morning with a loose powder and a fluffy brush and blot shine during the day with a blotting pick, e.g. blotting papers, a blotting sponge like BeautyBlender's Blotterazzi, or a pressed powder (easy on the pressed powder, as too many touchups will defeat the purpose of a skin-like finish). A pressed powder can also be used to lightly set your makeup with a large powder brush or applied with a sponge to add more coverage. Translucent powders, available in pressed or loose formulations are also good for touchups. When using these colorless powders, take care not to apply too much or fail to blend them well, because if you don't, they will give off a chalky cast on brown skin. They will also give you that dreaded look known as FLASHBACK because the light from a camera flash is known to bounce off the ingredients in these powders.

"I always like skin to look luminous, especially on women who are older, so I only powder the T-zone with a large fluffy brush so it doesn't look too made up," says Garnes, who's known for her classically beautiful faces on the red carpet and on TV. There are always exceptions, but the rule of thumb among the pros is that the powderful move now is not about mattifying the entire face but keeping it vibrant and alive. Besides, as Acey says, "you don't want to look casket-sharp!" Enough said.

Beauty Box: Powder

Whether pressed or loose, makeup always lasts longer when powder is in the mix.

- **Pressed:** Provides medium coverage; zaps shine.
- **Loose:** Offers light coverage; sets foundation; zaps shine.

Shopping Cart
Now that you know how you want to "powder-forward," here are some great picks to choose from.

- Clinique Stay-Matte Sheer Pressed Powder

- Jay Manuel Beauty Luxe Powder
- Iman Cosmetics Perfect Response Oil Blotting Powder
- Ben Nye Classic Translucent Face Powder
- Black Opal Deluxe Finishing Powder

---

66 **M**ost women are usually about one or two products shy of experiencing the results they want to achieve. Think of it like a recipe—if you make a cake and leave out one or two of the ingredients, it's not going to rise."

—Sam Fine, celebrity makeup artist

Bronzer Lust

There's nothing like a good bronzer to perk up a sallow complexion with a warm, sun-kissed glow. Whether you choose a lotion, a cream, or a powder, you can look fresh from the shores of a sunny isle in seconds, but here is where it can get challenging: picking the right shade. When shopping bronzer think: What's my best sun-warmed look? Then make it your goal to mimic that. Avoid products that are too red (disastrous) or muddy (hard, fake, and, worst of all, AGING!) or that have large shimmer pigments as they look totally unnatural, utterly cheap, and if you get fillers, they make you look puffy. Not good! Now, that aside, keep an open mind: your best bronzer could be a pressed powder, so don't get hung up on the label or the purpose. It could be a tinted moisturizer or a weightless liquid foundation where a pea-size amount applied with a foundation brush or a blender sponge gets you the results you want. It might be a bronzing powder that allows you to layer color with a large powder brush or a bronzing lotion that you mix in your hand with your moisturizer and apply so you get the most natural finish. So think light, think pretty, and go easy. Remember, you want to look like you've been sun-kissed, not sunbaked!

Blush Life

I learned the ins and outs of makeup from the best, beginning with my mother, who was a celebrity makeup artist, as well as the likes of Reggie Wells, Fran Cooper, Sam Fine, Jay Manuel, the late Roxanna Floyd, and Kevyn Aucoin, along with others whom I watched work with makeup in the most visionary ways. One pick they never skimped on was *blush*, and to this day it is such a versatile player that I say, "Don't leave home without working some element of it!" Now before you gasp, forget the old notions of those burgundy-hued standouts that make one look like a '70s makeup ad and rethink it as a luminous warming hue that adds tone and a little dimension to your look to keep you from looking flat. "With new technology came a movement that puts diffusing, low-level pearls into blush to make it glow, so now you're not only getting color you're getting a bit of shimmer," Fine notes, reminding us that it's not so Raggedy Ann: "Now it's about flush and glow." This is the modernity in makeup that continues the harmony of a skin-like finish, making it easier to select shades and textures that are synergistic with your base picks. Many powder blush compacts offer both a matte and a complementary shimmer alongside it. This combination makes the concept of "blush" more palatable and opens up your category of choices as well as your thinking beyond pink, orange, or burgundy cheeks. Formulas are also more sheer and blendable now and thus easier to control. Your range of cheek options also include great sticks, crayons, and creams that merge seamlessly with your skin. Oftentimes you'll also find bronzing creams, powders, or sticks the perfect echo as well. If you're fair, keep your choices soft, simple, and oh-so-sheer by selecting nudes with a hint of pink or peach to achieve what makeup artists refer to as a "healthy appeal." If you fall into the medium range, keep your choices deliberately warm, and feel free to mix in or sweep over a hint of bronze or apricot-gold so it looks fresh. If you're of a deeper hue, avoid matte, muddy shades like the plague, and keep it warm with a luminous orange like Nars Taj Mahal or a brick like MAC's Raizin, or have no fear and look to a browned rose like MAC's Pinch Me. I've been known to use a great eyeshadow in, say, a rhubarb or magenta. So when you're hitting the counters and aisles, shop hues that look great on you. Many makeup artists shop nontraditional products to add color, especially on us, where the nuances make all the difference in the world. So keep an open mind. Look for game-changing hues and smart picks that allow you the kind of versatility that ensures your best look.

Lashes: Fringe Benefits

Whenever I sit for makeup, the conversation always comes to a discussion on eyes and the look of the day. Without question, the eyes have it, as they punctuate your look unlike any other feature, which is why I always cut to the chase and ask, "What lash are we doing?" For TV, artists always like a good strip lash, maybe two (for real!), so the eyes have real depth and are utterly glamorous. Believe it or not, with the right lash—and an invisible strip—it never looks over the top. On my own, a great strip it is, and I have fun with a variety of styles. I've nailed the application down to a quick snap with a 5x magnifying mirror, lighted tweezers, and Duo Brush On Adhesive, which features an ultrathin brush for precise placement. I have an on-again, off-again affair with lash extensions because while they do simplify your life, survive many a spin class, and make for pretty eyes, they can weaken and cause breakage of your natural lashes, and if your lashes are fine like mine, that's a certainty. It takes anywhere from one to six months for your lashes to grow back, and that means sometimes they're not ready when you are! So plan your lash appointments accordingly.

Now as for the subject of mascara, clever packaging is fine, but I want you to know what's in it for you. In other words, how will it impact your style? And here you want a payoff that counts. When I take those all-important "lash breaks," I don't want to feel like something's missing, so the first thing I reach for is a lash booster when my fine short lashes need thickening. Next it's a few coats of a thickening mascara (allowing each coat to dry a little in between) so I get the lush effect I'm looking for. Here, too, you'll want to keep a keen eye on depth of color, what the brush looks like, how much product it deposits, *and* if it's buildable without clumping, and a lot of drugstore brands not only fit the bill, they are amazing. Anything that has to be pumped is a pass: the product performance should be so stellar that it allows you to drag the wand slowly from the base to the tips on the underside of your lashes (moving side to side, which also lifts lashes for a wide-eye effect), then comb through on top so that the results meet your expectations. I reserve the use of waterproof mascara for long days in humid climates, other gals use them on their wedding day when tears are sure to be shed. The rule of thumb here is this: avoid making them your mainstay as they take a minute to remove and experts say some formulas can be drying.

Shopping Cart

Up your lash game and create major effects with these wand-wonders!
- **Volume:** Urban Decay Perversion Mascara.
- **Lengthening:** MAC False Lashes.
- **Volume and length:** CoverGirl LashBlast Fusion Mascara.
- **Waterproof:** Lancôme Hypnôse Waterproof Custom Volume Mascara.
- **Sensitive eyes:** Almay One Coat Thickening Mascara.
- **Lash booster:** L'Oréal Voluminous Lash Primer.
- **Lower lashes:** Clinique Bottom Lash Mascara.

Whatever your makeup budget, know that there's no need to turn in your "glam pass." Just grab a cute roomy tote (Queens don't do plastic bags!) and hit the drugstore for those directional picks waiting for someone like you who's in the know about what works!

Mikki-ism

Line Up

A vivid liner, whether pencil, powder, liquid, or felt-tip, is an utterly chic way to make a statement. I love a bold stroke of color on bare lids framed by wispy lashes or a hint on the inner corner of a smoky eye coupled with sweeps of a lush black mascara. Think electric blue, parrot green, vibrant purple, or lush teal, and make an impact. Inky blues and rich black—especially smoky black pencils or gel liners with a hint of shimmer—ignite the eyes and in my book are mercurial madness! Delivery forms are a matter of preference, as it's really about what allows you the most control, staying power, and, if you're that doll, versatility.

Know Your Textures

- **Pencil:** Imparts a strong, opaque line.
- **Liquid:** Applied with a brush; gives a bold, matte, or shiny finish.
- **Felt-tip:** Available in thick or fine tips; gives matte definition with the application ease of a marker.
- **Crayon:** Creamier in texture than their slim counterparts; doubles as a liner or shadow.
- **Gel:** Concentrated color, matte finish.

Don't date yourself: Never, ever match makeup to your clothes. Makeup should complement, not match. Make it count!

Mikki-ism

Shadow Works: Throw Shade

As we see, oil is the enemy of a great look, so prepping is step one. Given our many skin tones, it's also important to use a primer that creates an opaque canvas to get the best color payoff from your eyeshadow, especially when using brands that aren't as pigmented. "Eyeshadows are hit-or-miss, and I find the more expensive brands have stronger pigments and you don't have to use as much to get the look you're going for," notes Acey. This is where a primer becomes a time-saver and a resolution when you've purchased what appeared to be a fabulous color in store, only to find that it doesn't pay off when you get home. As Acey notes, "You don't have time to put on sixteen layers of shadow just to make it look the same as it does in the package." Fine, who's been behind the scenes in product development with both mass and prestige brands, says, "When it comes to color and formula, it's not so specific that one brand is superior and another brand is inferior. It's that the technology isn't a part of some of the mass brands because they cost more money." On the other hand, if you're the doll who likes a hint of color, then your best bet is a sheer primer that checks creasing while allowing your skin to show through.

Defining a Look

Many say the eyes are the window to the soul. Well, if we're talking revelations, then they're the perfect play space to express yourself and have fun with your beauty. It's so not about getting stuck in a rut and trying to get the same look right every time. Where's the creativity in that? It's not a uniform, after all. It's makeup! I love how actress Lupita Nyong'o switches up her look. Whether she's working a deliberate sweep of color or "color blocking" that sees the chocolate beauty in a bright green liner on her upper lash line and a lush cobalt blue on the lower lash line with wispy lashes or a sheer wash of a bronzy metallic punctuated with black liner, she fearlessly moves her look forward every time I see her. I also love seeing Solange Knowles, whose fierce sense of self sees her tapping into all her options in color as well as metallics, and not just the traditional picks but hues like orange and platinum with a see-through prettiness that's so eye-catching. I knew she was a beauty girl to watch from the time I met her backstage as a young teen at a Destiny's Child performance. Look, with a mother as a makeup artist, I practically grew up backstage, where makeup was part of the magical art of being a woman. I came through the era of Diana Ross and the Supremes, and no one served a look on *The Ed Sullivan Show* like those divas! Ms. Ross knew her beauty so well that when I worked with her on her first *Essence* cover in 1982, she did her own makeup, by choice! In fact, in 2005 MAC Cosmetics named Ross as its *Beauty Icon* to represent a new collection named after the Super Star and it featured the most amazing hues. No surprise there, women like Ross, and those who came before her, inspired us with their approach to makeup before they had the options in color, let alone the range of neutrals that we have today, but they mixed and created their look both on and off duty to the thrill of us all. And that's the point: it's about defining a look and enjoying the process, and if not now, when? Don't see it as a challenge. See it as an opportunity and take a "why not?" approach, and if you decide that eye makeup or makeup period isn't for you, so what? You're fine whether you ever wear makeup or not, but given the many fresh options in hues and textures that are finally available for us, I think you should at least know.

Beauty Box
Shadow Works: Know Your Textures

- **Pressed powders:** Sheer to opaque finish.
- **Loose powders:** Sheer finish.
- **Creams:** Buildable finish.
- **Crayons:** Sheer to opaque finish.

Be creative. Find your best lip hue and glam it overtime! Gloss it, matte it, and, by all means, paint it to perfection.

Mikki-ism

Pout Perfection

The lives of women of color have evolved so much. There was a time when full lips weren't thought of as beautiful in America, yet when I was a beauty director, the women with full lips were my muses—the fuller, the better. When I worked with Naomi Campbell for her first *Essence* cover, she was only fifteen at the time and had only been photographed in Europe with nude lips. I had makeup artist Reggie Wells paint every inch of her gorgeous pillowy lips in a velvet red that you had to deal with. It wasn't because red lips were trending; it was because her *lips* took red to a fever pitch! Fast-forward to the present, I can tell you when I see women like Kerry Washington, Estelle, Meagan Good, or designer muse Aya Jones (who descended from the Ivory Coast and turned the fashion world upside down) in bold red lips or a steamy gloss infused with shimmer, I'm over the moon because change was a long time coming. Whether you're a red-lip muse, a *fuchsia*-nista fave, an in-the-bare doll, or one who's "in deep," in that you favor midnight blues and licorice blacks—whatever you prefer, be deliberate, all shades, all sizes, and embrace what's yours. Never bow out of the joy of celebrating your beauty, *all* of your beauty.

The Right Buff

Politics and perceptions aside, all hues and textures look best on lips that are well cared for. Make a weekly scrub with a washcloth, soft toothbrush, or an exfoliating lip product like Bliss Fabulips Sugar Lip Scrub part of your regimen. Religiously using an emollient that softens and seals in hydration by night and a smoothing lip balm under your lip pick by day will complement your efforts. If your lips are uneven in tone, use a depigmentation balm at night and an opaque lip primer under your lipstick to create an even canvas. If fine lines, which can destroy a matte lip, are a concern, get a lip treatment that has skin-smoothing peptides like Peter Thomas Roth Un-Wrinkle Lip or Murad Rapid Collagen Infusion for Lips.

Buildup

The real purpose of a lip liner is to define your natural lip line and prevent lipstick from bleeding. Contrary to popular belief, you do not need to buy lip pencils in the various shades of the lipsticks you wear. Simply choose a shade close to the tone of your lips. I find a lip liner to be an essential component of successfully working a nude lip, particularly if it's a matte lipstick, as without this it will get lost. Lip liners can also play a role in intensifying your lip color. For example, if you wish to wish to add depth to a soft red basing your lips with a burgundy pencil will give it new dimension.

You Better Work!
Chic Strategies for the Cool in You

Compact Beauty

When I was a child, my mother always had the most beautiful mirrored compacts. As a makeup artist who traveled globally, my mother had the most amazing beauty finds in general, from the enchanting little drams of foundation that matched her rich brown skin long before she could buy the same here in the States, to handheld mirrors, powder puffs, and more. However, it was the mirrored compacts that graced her dresser and accompanied her on the most important occasions that thrilled me, and thus my love of these beauty jewels was born. I'm always on the lookout for a great compact and never resist my urges for the sublime. You can scour vintage shops, department stores, old-world pharmacies, and the internet for the prettiest finds one can imagine. Sometimes I come across a great powder compact made especially to hold loose powder, complete with a mesh veil, and I'm smitten! Depending on your skin tone, you can also find beautiful compacts at department store cosmetic counters that contain translucent powder; however, for brown girls like me, they tend to leave an unnatural cast that, to put it mildly, makes me look as though I'm about to leave here! Nevertheless, I think every gal should have at least one compact mirror to check her image in and declare herself fabulous. Click.

Heat Wave

When the heat is on, nothing makes for a more sizzling beauty moment than glowing skin and a single punch of color! Adding a drop of an illuminator to your foundation is all it takes for a fresh, sun-kissed radiance that you'll want to work again and again. When paired with a juicy orange on the lips and a few sweeps of black mascara, you'll be so there.

Radiant Picks
- Giorgio Armani Maestro Liquid Summer
- Le Métier de Beauté Bella Bronzer Liquid Illuminator
- Nars Illuminator

Punch Works
- Maybelline Color Sensational Vivids Lipcolor in Electric Orange
- Revlon Colorburst Matte Balm in Audacious

- MAC Cosmetics Sheen Supreme in Sweet Grenadine
- Marc Jacobs Kiss Pop Lipstick in Pop Rock
- Jay Manuel Beauty The Ultimate Lipstick in MILF

Pretty Fresh

What's big on style, sophistication, and service? Why, a fabulous handheld fan of course! And you, my dear, should have at least one for those times when you're in a crowd, stepping out on a hot day, or when you get a little steam of your own making. Trust me, a Queen is always prepared for any situation that presents itself. Don't even think about relying on a tissue. Tissues are so not it. They leave residue, absorb makeup, fall apart, and need to be discarded. I say look for those that speak to your personal style, and keep one in your bag for any and all occasions where you need to keep cool. Those that have a little weight are not only the most effective but also the most resilient. So whether you find yours on the internet or hit the best gift shops, do pick up your most stylish bet for keeping cool on the go. Who says we can't style at every turn?

Nitty-Gritty

Spring cleaning? Don't forget your makeup stash. Though makeup doesn't come with an expiration date, it certainly does have a shelf life. It's tempting to hold onto your faves, especially those that have been discontinued, yet there comes a point when you just have to let go since over time makeup becomes grounds for bacteria. So be on it: immediately discard any makeup that is broken or cracked (powders) missing a lid, smells acrid, or has separated. And contrary to belief, don't store your makeup in the bathroom, where heat and humidity are known to promote the growth of mold and yeast; instead, stash your makeup in a cool, dry place, perhaps in a metal storage bin in your bedroom, to prolong its use. I keep my picks in my vanity, which has convenient storage spaces and drawers. Housekeeping aside, keep in mind the basics on makeup shelf life:

- **Liquid foundation:** One year (if not stored in direct sunlight).

- **Face powder:** Up to two years.
- **Powder blush:** Up to two years—but if the texture hardens or has oil slicks/spots and the color can't be accessed, toss it.
- **Concealers:** Six months.
- **Cream blush:** One year.
- **Eyeshadow:** Six months to a year.
- **Mascara, eyeliner:** Two to three months.
- **Lipstick:** Up to two years (once it hardens and the color won't budge, toss).
- **Lip gloss:** Up to two years.

Tighten Up

Do hit cosmetic counters that allow you to put together your own capsulized collection of hues and textures for eyes, cheeks, and lips in a single compact. Too haute to miss: Bobbi Brown, Trish McEvoy, and MAC (freestanding stores only). The nicety here is you can snap your finds out and replace them as often as you like. Now there's a cool experience.

Evening Perk-Up

I used to love slipping into Sam Fine's chair for a makeup cleanup before heading out to a gala. After many lessons, I learned how to clean up well myself! The trick is to focus on products and techniques that refresh your day makeup and allow you to take it to the next level without looking "stale." First, don't even think about reapplying your foundation unless you're going to cleanse it off and start all over again! Instead, blot skin with blotting paper to absorb any oil in the T-zone. Then spritz your skin with a face mist to rehydrate and refresh. Remove your lipstick with a cleansing remover wipe so you don't dry your lips out. Touch up your blush, dust powder in the T-zone, and add a sweep of bronzer on your cheekbones. Apply eyeliner on your upper lash line; using an eyeshadow stick, add a hint of a neutral metallic hue on your lids. Next, apply mascara or a light, feathery lash. Apply lip primer/balm and complete the look with a fab matte lipstick or a sensuous gloss.

Take Five

When you've got to dash, whether to work, a meeting, or a last-minute invitation, creating a fresh look in five minutes is easy with the right picks and techniques, so don't overthink it. Besides, when you know your face, you can achieve a great look with a minimal amount of products. Let's go:

- Apply a tinted moisturizer (you can create your own using a couple of drops of liquid makeup and your moisturizer) or CC cream, and blend using a large sponge; if you need coverage, use stick foundation where needed and again blend with a sponge so the look is seamless.
- Using a multipurpose pick like a large crayon, apply color to your cheeks and lips; blend the color out on your cheeks with a sponge and blend on lips using a lip brush.
- Dust your T-zone with powder.
- Sweep on mascara, and brush and fill in brows.

Time to spare? Line eyes and sweep on a sheer browned shadow, or go for the impact of a striking matte lip, which makes a nice contrast against fresh "skin."

On a hot day, I want this: a chilled drink, a fabulous fan, a grill that I don't have to man, and to look cool and lovely! Waterproof makeup, anyone?

Mikki-ism

Summer-Night Style

Whether you're headed to a glamorous poolside gathering or dinner under the stars, keep your look modern and effortless. I love keeping cool while turning up in heat-wave friendly dresses in Acapulco-inspired hues. On the beauty front, think "clean glamour," and consider shading eyes in soft desert tones so as not to compete, and use waterproof liner and mascara; then imagine a bold, matte cherry or a zesty orange glossed lip, even a cool matte fuchsia thrilling a red dress to madness! Talk about style nailed to the point.

Smoke Signals

Intrigue comes in many forms, but one that always heats up a look is a smoky eye paired with a lush nude lip. Whether you ignite your eyes in cool tones like inky deeps, woody browns, or stormy grays or those that are warm like molasses, rich chocolates, or coffee browns, when paired with a nude lip, it never disappoints. Here's the thing, though: choose your lip pick from soft satins, sheers, or gloss, but be careful with mattes. Only the smoothest lips need apply! Why? Matte nudes showcase everything, including that which you'd prefer not to.

All Fired Up!

Be it a directional matte, a sophisticated satin, or a sensuous sheer, I find nothing punctuates a look and kicks it into iconic status like the perfect red lip. Why not electrify your style and put spring fever on overdrive with a fabulous, cannot-be-ignored red? It's an utterly fast way to pull a look together as it couldn't be simpler than working a seemingly bare skin finish (think a BB cream: a little coverage but lighter than foundation, with skin care benefits) with well-groomed brows, coats of a lash-boosting mascara, and pairing it all with a divine crimson hue. Now you may be asking, how do I choose my perfect red? The so-called rules vary as skin tone, hair color, and even the color of your eyes play a role. I say "so-called," as I've seen style mavens who break them with panache and fiercely make their own rules. However, when in doubt, you can't go wrong with the following cheat sheet: A true red (tomato) is a glamorous basic and is generally flattering on most beauties, from fair to deep. Ditto for most blue-based reds, albeit a little more intense for those on the fairer end of the color spectrum, but if you're a fair and fearless one like actresses Paula Patton or Grace Byers, you'll work it! And here's the big beauty bonus: bold, blue-based red lip shades also make your pearly whites gleam in nanoseconds. A fiery orange red is totally sexy on browned beauties like Queen Latifah or Janelle Monáe. Browned reds, well, honestly, they can be a little tricky, but on medium-brown skin tones like Gabrielle Union's and Iman's, they work well—as makeup artist Sam Fine says, they "jump off the skin just enough for you to read it." Whatever red you choose, be sure to set it off with ultrasmooth lips and a primer to make it last. See you on Instagram looking amazing!

Blue-Chip Reds to Bag

1 MAC Cosmetics Lipstick in Ruby Woo
2 Kevyn Aucoin Expert Lip Color in Carliana
3 Tom Ford Lip Color in Cherry Lush
4 Nars Semi-Matte Lipstick in Heat Wave
5 Bobbi Brown Creamy Matte Lip Color in Red Carpet

Thrifty Business

Don't you just love a beauty bargain? Ditto! I hit drugstores and beauty supply centers everywhere in search of a great steal. I think that beauty is centered in discovery, and so I'm always on the lookout for something different. What it taught me is this: makeup trends come and go, but if you have a good eye, you can work a $5 lipstick just as well as one that costs $15. So when it comes to great finds and brag-worthy prices, here are five glam picks that you can bank on for under $10:

1 Red lipstick
2 Black eyeliner
3 Mascara
4 Bronzer
5 Pressed powder

Survival of the Chicest

Don't let carry-on restrictions cramp your style and alter your stash of beauty must-haves. With a cleverly packed bag, you can have not only what you need but also a few extras—hello! Here's how it's done:

- Make sure your carry-on bag has lots of pockets for things like hand cream and miniature beauty product tubes, which are always fine to take on board.
- Hit your favorite beauty counters for deluxe travel-size versions of your favorite liquid skin care picks that'll fit that quart-size bag requirement.
- Don't miss out on department store GWPs (gifts with purchase), as more often than not, they come with travel-size picks and a cosmetic or tote bag as well.
- Shop the travel aisle in drugstores for minis. You'll find everything there from your favorite antiperspirant to petroleum jelly.
- Take a roller-ball version of your fragrance fave instead of a spray.
- Decant, decant, decant anything that you can't live without.

In-Flight Beauty

I've gotten so used to hopping on a plane that it's like getting on the bus, and to keep my life and my look intact, I keep a packing list on the computer and a beauty kit that's ready to go. Flying high at thirty-seven thousand feet isn't as glamorous as it sounds, no matter where you're headed. It's a "beauty hurdle" because, as we know, you get dehydrated, your circulation suffers, and invisible germs abound! Here are a few practices I've found that help one arrive looking refreshed:

- Hydration is the objective: always fly in a hydrating serum that contains moisture-retaining hyaluronic acid, moisturizer with SPF, and lots of hand cream. It's important to keep your skin protected as you're even closer to the sun's damaging rays when flying, so don't forget this! Just before landing, I refresh with a spritz of Caudalie Beauty Elixir, a facial mist that's part serum and part toner, with active plant ingredients to boost radiance. I also add a hydrating serum to my hair on long-haul flights to keep it shiny and sleek because I don't want to look as if I got lost in a desert.

- To master a rested look adding a little definition to your eyes makes all the difference. I rely on a long-wearing eye pencil, be it a fine one for lining or a crayon that I can smudge to give my eyes a little depth, and a thickening mascara (or, if headed to a meeting, a light lash like Ardell 110).

On-the-Go

When it comes to long days and festive nights, it's all about having those essentials that keep pace with your lifestyle. I've found that dazzling from a.m. to p.m. calls for a short list of the best beauty buys that help you work overtime. In makeup: it's a great time to carry the perfect multitasking face palette and mini-brushes in your bag. On the scent trek: travel light and look to roller-balls or sample-size sprays of your favorite fragrance for touch-ups. In hair: think sample-size stylers, perhaps travel tools, and maybe even a crown jewel like a stoned ponytail holder, a clip or even a brooch for a quick switch! My layered do calls for a dry shampoo to refresh, a glossing cream for smoothing and catching flyaways, and a compact brush with a mirror. Depending on your look and texture, yours might call for a different set of staples. The takeaway: whether you're touching up at the office or on the go, always have what you need on hand to style.

Notes to Self...

Notes to Self...

4

Hands, Nails,
and Footnotes

Technology has brought us a long way from the days when a handful of products and a few basic services were all there was to be had for sister-women. In the area of what I call "the Communicators," a.k.a. our hands, nails, and feet, we now have pharmaceutical change agents to retexturize skin to a previously unattainable level of softness, lasers that address pigmentary concerns, and age-defying techniques at the hands of pros who understand what that means to us. We can step into the salon or hit beauty destinations for the chicest finds and be the trendsetters that we are due to the revolution in color, formulations, and new age tools. Yet as important as it is to have all the best style and improvement options at our fingertips, a strong DIY strategy is still important.

Your hands, nails, and feet are your major players, and in order for them to serve you well, let alone *speak* well of you, you must give them the TLC they deserve. Yours Truly loves to beat it into the best chairs in the business for a mani-pedi, but I'm just as driven about care on the home front. Like those of any busy wife/mother/everywoman, my hands and nails suffer from everything one can think of, from just being on-duty to environmental exposure. And my feet, well, that's a whole other tale of perilous high heels, pointy toes, and long hours on the go that often have them crying for a little fashion mercy! So much for fun, right? Truth is, a lot more goes into the maintenance picture for us brown-skin beauties who never skip a beat on the style front. It calls for a regimen that treats matters like hyperpigmentation and texture concerns and protects our hands, nails, and feet against the rigors of a demanding lifestyle and the changes that take place as we age.

AFFIRMATION

Shake the expected and push for the possibilities!

Hands Down

The real news is this: you should be caring for the skin on your hands much like you do the skin on your face. "Most of us couldn't leave the bathroom after washing our face without putting on a moisturizer. How many times do we wash our hands and not put on a moisturizer?" says Deborah Lippmann, founder and creative director of her own signature nail line. Our hands tend to be much drier due to a lack of oil glands, so hydration is essential. To protect them with a glove-like barrier, turn to noteworthy basics like hand creams that contain such hydrating ingredients as glycerin, keratin, ceramides, and hyaluronic acid. What's also seriously recommended is incorporating the use of a hand cream with sunscreen. Though the melanin in our skin does play a photo-protective role, using a hand cream with an SPF of 15 or above is important, especially if you tend to have any unevenness or hyperpigmented areas like dark knuckles. When you think about it, our hands are constantly exposed. Even when driving, your hands are what's catching the sun's rays. And though the danger debate continues over UV lights used during gel manicures, Lippmann suggests applying a hand cream with SPF before you put your hands in the machine. "Some salons have fingerless gloves to protect you from the light, so why take the chance without protecting yourself?" Lippmann asks.

I'm all about rituals at night as I see this as the time for the Queen to restore herself. Most of the hand models in the business take extra care of their hands at night because their hands are a precious commodity. You can call on some of the same practices they do, like massaging your hands on a nightly basis with warm coconut oil or a nutrient-rich moisturizer or serum with treatment benefits that specifically address your concerns. Some hand models go a step further, slathering their hands with their treatment of choice and sleeping in a pair of thin cotton gloves.

Keeping hands soft, smooth, and even also calls for exfoliating dead skin. This can be done manually with a commercial hand scrub, or you can make your own by combining baby or almond oil and sea salt or fine Himalayan pink salt—my fave (I suggest keeping this on your kitchen or bathroom sink so you'll be reminded to dip in)— which will polish skin without stripping it dry. Today's chemical exfoliants also help speed up the sloughing action, and ingredients like glycolic and lactic acids leave skin super smooth. "Glycolic acid is a great exfoliating agent that peels away the dead skin cells that accumulate on the hands," says NYC dermatologist Howard Sobel, who recommends incorporating it with hydrating scrubbing beads as an effective retexturizer. Hand creams that contain glycolic or alpha hydroxy acid, both widely available ingredients in commercial formulas, represent another way to reveal soft, smooth skin. Exfoliation is also effective for treating tough spots such as rough knuckles and any hyperpigmentation (an all-too-common complaint for chocolate beauties) as it not only eliminates dead skin cells but also allows for treatments that address discoloration, such as those containing ingredients like hydroquinone, ferulic acid, or arbutin, to penetrate deeper and faster. If you find fading dark knuckles with over-the-counter products problematic, don't hesitate to see a dermatologist who can recommend a prescriptive formulation or take treating the area a step further. "This is where we do chemical peels and lasers to help break up the pigment," says NYC dermatologist Dr. Fran Cook-Bolden, who adds, "Lasers like the Nd:YAG have been proven very effective (even for melasma, which is very tough to treat, because heat can make melasma worse) for us." When laser therapy is done on low settings and multiple passes in the hands of an expert who's familiar with skin of color, it does a great job at breaking up resistant hyperpigmentation.

Keeping It Real

The skin located on the top of the hands is very fragile and thin and is constantly exposed to drastic climate changes (e.g., sunlight, dry/cold air, etc.), all of which impact the skin. When you couple this with the way we age (loss of volume and firmness and increased dryness), you can see why the true sign of one's age can be guesstimated by a glance at the hands. I say take matters into your own hands (pun intended) and start treating them with targeted hand care and, at the first sign of aging, ingredients that go beyond pampering them. "Retinol works the same for hands as it does for the face by activating the collagen and elastin production response," says Dr. Sobel. This produces younger-looking skin. What also produces more youthful hands are injectables, and nowadays dermatologists are using fillers like Sculptra to enhance volume and coupling them with skin care products containing antioxidants like green tea and vitamin C because they help to reverse the damage that free radicals do to the skin in breaking down collagen.

Dividing Lines

Veins have a way of sneaking up on you and taking center stage on the back of your hands due to various reasons like the normal aging process, which causes skin to lose its volume and elasticity; veins are also exacerbated by exercise, which causes the blood pressure in the arteries to increase, forcing blood to pool around your muscles and in turn push your veins toward the skin's surface. The good news is you don't have to live with them. There are minimally invasive procedures like fillers that will restore your look without any downtime. Though fillers are only a temporary fix (they last up to nine months) they do "plump" up the skin and eliminate the look of bulging veins that appear as one ages.

Stop the Madness

No matter how tempting it is, please don't cut your cuticles or let anyone else "surgical style" them! "The only part of the cuticle that should ever be nipped are hangnails," says Lippmann. Cuticles are living tissue, and they need pampering, not *cutting*, to stay smooth. Besides, they're there to protect you, so you must let them do their job and guard your nails from incoming bacteria. Just say no, drop the clippers, and look to today's tech-smart product solutions to keep your cuticles smooth and tight. I thought I would need a twelve-step program to stop having my cuticles cut at the salon, but I found cuticle-specific treatments with exfoliating ingredients will smooth the cuticles (when used religiously) and prevent buildup. "Most of our cuticle problems are due to the fact that we don't remember we need to exfoliate our cuticles," adds Lippmann. The nail pro says many salons put on cuticle oil and push the cuticles back, but "that's like putting a serum on your face and rubbing it and hoping it will exfoliate, and it won't," she explains. It's not about a quick cosmetic fix, but rather using a cuticle *remover* and pushing the cuticles back as part of a weekly manicure.

Cutting your cuticles will also cause them to peel, and if you've ever experienced this, you know it's quite painful. When this happens, Lippmann offers this healing solution: "Gently exfoliate using a hand scrub and a cuticle remover to dissolve the excess skin, and follow with moisture and more moisture!" I avoid this painful scenario by working a hydrating hand cream on my cuticles by day when the real damage is done and using a cuticle oil by night. Treats like these will keep yours smooth, pretty, and trim-free, too.

66 **Y**our nails are your greeters and your hands say
a lot about you. I don't think you have to wear
polish, but you have to be polished."

—Deborah Lippmann

Take Care

According to celebrity manicurist Lisa Logan, "everything starts with
the foundation, and if the end results are going to be beautiful, you
need a strong healthy nail." While the market is flooded with nail
strengtheners and products claiming to give you resilient nails, there's
no skipping out on good nutrition as it plays a direct role in *growing* strong healthy nails to begin with. Getting enough protein is key.
"Protein in the diet not only helps to strengthen nails, which are made
of protein themselves," says the woman known as America's nutrition
coach, Dr. Ro, "but the calcium in protein sources like low-fat cheese,
yogurt, and dairy also help."

When it comes to external care, nurturing your nails is another
way of honoring yourself and celebrating your beauty, and whether
you place yourself in the hands of a pro or turn out your own perfect ten, it's time worth devoting to yourself, totally uninterrupted. I
always say whatever you put into an experience is what you get out of
it. The same holds true for your nails. Self-maintenance is an essential
form of preservation that you don't want to cut short, so before you
think color, shape, length, or any style moves, first think nail care and
identify those practices that will support strong, healthy, and flexible
nails. Logan, whose clients include Mary J. Blige, Queen Latifah, and
Taraji P. Henson, says, "Self-maintenance is preservation, and when
done properly, it makes for less work at your nail appointments and
helps preserve your manicure." It's really about covering your bases
no matter how you style, color or not. This is where coatings, as in

base and top coats, play a significant role. Base coats not only provide a foundation for your polish to adhere to but also prime, treat, and, where necessary, strengthen your nails. Top coats add high shine and a protective finish. If you're not a fan of polish, Dr. Suzanne Levine, of Institute Beauté in NYC, recommends keeping your natural nail healthy and bright by mixing baking soda and hydrogen peroxide into a paste and scrubbing your nails gently with a toothbrush twice a week. Buffing is another good practice for your natural nail as it improves circulation and keeps nails strong, healthy, and smooth. Above all, Lippmann says, "your nails should be groomed, filed, and all the same length."

Oddly enough, the things we take for granted are what can affect the strength of our nails, as well as the length of a manicure, the most. Take, for example, soaking nails in water. This is a common practice but a real no-no because water penetrates the nails, weakens them, and compromises the length of your manicure. Think about it: You wouldn't do the dishes without rubber gloves for the same reason, right? I say try a warm cream soak instead (simply heat hand cream in the microwave) and you'll see the difference.

The shape of your nails and how they are filed also plays a role. Always file nails gently in one direction as filing them back and forth will weaken them. When it comes to shape, Lippmann maintains that it's about filing up the sidewall of the nail so it remains straight and wide (not curved) so that the base remains strong. "Where the nail turns white is called the 'free edge'—this is the stress point of your nails and where breakage occurs," she explains. Shaping your nails just past the point where the free edge begins makes for a stronger nail. Keep in mind that while nail strengtheners can help, consistent use of a nourishing hand cream to keep them hydrated will play a role as well, as a lack of moisture can also make nails susceptible to splitting or peeling.

You can also nail your look and prevent damage by avoiding the following culprits:

- Acetone removers and hair products that contain alcohol: Extremely drying.

- Nail lacquers containing toluene and formaldehyde: Drying.

- Heavy-grit nail files: They act like sandpaper and will wear your nails down.

- Filing/sawing back and forth: Weakens nails.

- Quick-dry top coats: Shrink polish as they dry and cause polish to chip faster.

- Using your nails as tools: Weakens nails and invites breakage.

- Texting and typing with your nails: Leads to breakage.

Regardless of how you pick your paint, nail it!

Mikki-ism

Strokes of Genius

If a pro gel manicure isn't your thing, making that gorgeous DIY manicure last is something that's top of mind. Nowadays there are ways to duplicate salon effects at home, as gel manicure kits are becoming widely available; there are also gel polishes, of course, and even next-generation gel top coats that add longevity. If you are a gel devotee like Yours Truly, I know you love the instantly dry, no-chip, two-week finish, but do know that these advantages don't place one in the "maintenance-free zone." Regular care is a nonnegotiable, and in addition to your salon visits, be sure to protect your investment by incorporating the use of a protective top coat. "Think of this coating as the shield that keeps it all together and a valuable player that extends the life of your manicure," says Logan, who recommends touching up your nails with a top coat every three days after your manicure.

Snap to It

Think of your basic manicure as time for self—no phone, no distractions—just you, your thoughts, and the picks that make it happen.

- Gather your tools: nail brush, small bowl, emery board, buffing disc, pumice stick, orangewood stick, loose cotton (more absorbent than cotton balls), body scrub, shower gel, acetone-free polish remover, cuticle remover, hand towel, hand cream, base coat (for your nail type), polish, top coat.

- Prep: set up your space and lay out your tools and lacquers on the hand towel.

- Begin: saturate cotton with remover and remove all polish.

- Massage hands with your body scrub, then cleanse with a skin-softening shower gel.

- File nails gently in one direction into your preferred shape to prevent weakening them.

- Use the buffing disc lightly on the edges of your nails, and smooth any rough areas on the surface of the nails.

- Warm hand cream in a microwave.

- Apply cuticle remover and soak hands in hand cream.

- Remove excess hand cream, massage hands, and gently push back your cuticles with the pumice stick.

- Wrap cotton around the orangewood stick, dampen with remover, and wipe nail plate clean; also clean under the tips of your nails.

- Apply base coat, starting at the bottom center of the nail bed and extending to the tip. Repeat to complete the entire nail and ultimately continue until all nails are coated.

- Apply two coats of nail polish, allowing for a brief drying time in between the coats.

- Using the orangewood stick, remove any excess polish that may have seeped onto the cuticles.

- Apply top coat and allow it to dry completely.

Growth Strategies

I caution you against going by a "rule of thumb" when it comes to nail growth as it varies. Growth and retention are impacted by diet, vitamin deficiencies, medications, chemotherapy, and avoiding the culprits that can weaken your nails. What is essential for growing strong nails is eating a diet full of protein-rich foods and keeping your body hydrated to prevent brittleness. As for those supplements aimed at stimulating nail growth, experts like Dr. Richard K. Scher, clinical professor of dermatology at Weill Cornell Medicine, are cautious, noting that internalized supplements don't say "I'm going specifically to the nail plate." "If we had a product that could make the nails grow faster, that would be the equivalent of giving people younger nails," he concludes. What does impact the condition of your nails is biotin, in that it improves nail fragility and makes them less likely to split, crack, and peel, so it essentially helps preserve your nail plate.

Nude and Improved

Ballet-pink nude nails setting off a French manicure have long been a staple for the working set. I say: time to raise the barre and modernize your perfect ten. The definition of "nude" has changed, and bold white toppers are passé. Now nude nails with a degree of "next" are a lot more chic and utterly complementary: think minimalist classics like beige, greige (gray-beige), sandstone hues reminiscent of an island beach, and muted twilight hues like mauve. The best nudes are to your hands what fine lingerie is to your wardrobe—they complement and support your look—and the right hues make all the difference in the world. Nudes range from warm to cool in hue and vary in tone and depth. Whether you choose a soft sheer, an opaque cream, or a transparent shimmer, it's all about finding one that looks amazing on your skin. But beware of those that are so close to your skin tone that they make your hands look like paws or mannequin hands, a real no-no. Instead, work those that offer contrast and complement your skin and its undertones.

When it comes to modernizing the French manicure, think contrasting toppers of a different hue. "The update is it doesn't have to be tipped in white. You can take that template and add a different color to give it a pop or maybe subtle stones or try a half-moon," Logan says. It's about creating your own statement, so experiment and bring a fresh dash of cool to your take. Celebrity manicurist Deborah Lippmann, who's worked with such A-Listers as Academy Award–winning actress Lupita Nyong'o, favors "any color on the tip and any color on the nail that coordinates: red and pink, green and purple, a sheer base and a shimmer on the tip."

Though your style options on the French abound, the pros express that there is a right and a wrong way to wear it and agree that tips rendered in a straight white line more than a quarter-inch long fall into the latter category. "I like a French with a 'smile line,' otherwise known as a C-curve, so it's chic and classy," says Logan. Others frown on the square take bearing a large white band as it takes on the character of shovels—not a good look. "That's not chic. It should just be a sliver of white," Lippmann notes.

I remember the first time I worked with Erykah Badu. It was for the August 1997 cover of *Essence*, and as always, I brought along an array of on-trend nail hues to choose from. Individualist that she is, Badu chose several, with one hand in an olive green and the other hand completed with a different hue for each nail. It was a fast-forward move that exemplifies the way she sees herself and celebrates her style sensibility. Not one to wait for anything to come down the runway to validate her look, she's always been miles ahead.

I love a great nail conversation! Tell me a story, give me a visual, and slay me with a fabulous pattern, but please keep it chic. Island vistas and cheap prints work best on cosmetic bags!

Mikki-ism

cuticle remover, hydrating foot cream, orangewood stick, loose cotton, body scrub, shower gel, essential oils (optional), acetone-free polish remover, base coat, polish, and top coat.

- Prep: set up your space and lay out your tools and lacquers on the bath towel, and fill your basin with warm water, a few drops of an essential oil of your choice, and half a cup of milk or a mixture of Listerine and vinegar to soften dead skin.

- Remove your polish using an acetone-free polish remover.

- Soak feet for approximately ten minutes; then use your body scrub and exfoliate feet all over, rinse, remove, and pat dry.

- Hit heels and calluses with your foot file or pedi tool, and finish the process using the fine-grain section so that after you've removed the dead skin buildup, you refine the overall surface of your skin.

- Clip toenails straight across to prevent ingrown nails, and file nails using a coarse emery board. Smooth edges with a fine emery board.

- Follow by applying a cuticle remover and gently push back your cuticles.

- Buff the surface of your nail plate.

- Then treat feet to a hydrating mask by applying your foot cream. Place each foot in a plastic bag and wrap a hand towel around each, letting it remain on for five minutes.

⦿ Remove the bags and massage any residue from the cream into your skin. Put on your toe separators and clean nail beds using a cotton swab dampened with remover to make sure they are clean and dry.

⦿ Now you're ready to polish. Begin applying your base coat from the bottom center of the nail bed and complete the process by coating the entire nail. Follow with two coats of polish and your top coat.

Style and Substance

I've learned a few tricks of the trade over the years from the best in the business that allow me to work a smart balancing act without indulging in the popular injectables in use today to pad one's feet and lessen the impact of hot heels. I rely on gel pads to cushion my feet when on heel duty, and when doing red-carpet interviews, I call on Stiletto Rx (www.pillowsforyourfeet.com), a unique foot spray, developed by NYC podiatrist Dr. Suzanne Levine, that contains lidocaine to extend heel time. I'm not alone. A-listers and everyday divas all have their arsenal of sole savers that allow them to remain true to their Louboutins, Blahniks, and Choos. Now, you might think the former rely on their drivers and the latter work trainers on the go. Trust me, not so. Driving shoes only go so far, and the girls wouldn't be caught dead outside the gym in sneakers unless they are of an ilk meant for styling. More often than not, they switch out of foldable or stylish flats just before they hit their destination. Believe me, we all make these "Wonder Woman" moves, whether in the car or a hotel restroom, in order to preserve our feet in between life on demand!

Seriously, though, if you're a devoted heel wearer, experts recommend going a step further and invoking your own "boot camp" workout by doing exercises that will strengthen the muscles, tendons, and ligaments in your feet as well as your ankles, so get busy picking up marbles with your toes, tracing the alphabet with them, and rotating your ankles in circular motions several times a week. I also found out about the ProStretch Original Calf Stretcher (available at Amazon.com) from a physical therapist that's genius at releasing tight calves, and now I wouldn't be without it. Finally, I urge you to recognize that not all heels and materials are created equal, so balance the days when you're in stilettos against the days you're in wider heels, knowing that the wider the heel, the more comfortable the shoe. Understand that patents and some faux leathers can be killers, so skip the torment and choose soft materials whenever possible. Think fabric shoes, suedes, and soft leathers. And keep in mind that no matter how beloved, when shoes are too worn, they can no longer provide the support and cushioning your feet require and they'll do more harm than good.

Clearly sole survival calls for a plan of action; however, if you've tried your share of self-help options, know that you don't have to go it alone. Today great planning options are taking place in doctors' offices across the nation. One such option sees podiatrists incorporating the use of fillers with great success to restore volume and cushioning to the bottom of the foot. Why is this practice so popular now? "As we age, we lose padding (the layer of fat that lines your soles) on the bottom of the foot, and with the loss of padding, your four-inch heels become torture devices," notes Dr. Levine, who looks to Sculptra as a solution for her patients with this concern. A typical patient requires one to two syringes of the filler to treat the feet completely, and results generally last about a year. Costs vary depending on the provider, starting on average at $600, and can range from $450 to $550 per syringe. The procedure is said to be perfect for active professionals.

Word to the Wise
Your feet will grow and change shape over time due to the aging process, so it's a good idea to have them measured periodically to ensure

you're investing in shoes of the right size and width. When shopping, don't buy shoes early in the day, as you won't get an accurate fit. I confess, I'm sorry for every time that I ignored this rule! Also, err on the side of rounded toes whenever possible to alleviate bunions, which are exacerbated when toes are squeezed together by tight shoes with small toe boxes and pointy toes. Bunion surgery has its pros and cons, just like any other surgery, and recovery can take anywhere from six weeks to six months. The pros are that it can alleviate pain, improve physical activity, and improve the look of your feet. The cons are that bunion surgery has been associated with setbacks like unrelieved pain, reoccurrence of the bunion, and in some instances shoe restrictions for life. However, if you're experiencing pain that impacts the quality of your life, it's best to see a podiatrist or an orthopedic physician to discuss your best surgical options. Selecting the right surgeon is critical, so make sure your doctor is board-certified, experienced at performing bunion surgery, and, if possible, that this is their specialization, as not all surgeons are created equal and this is about more than your vanity!

Hammertoes (a contracture or bending deformity of one or both joints that occurs most frequently on the second toe) are another foot condition that you want to be proactive about as they usually get progressively worse over time if left untreated. The most common cause is a tendon imbalance, which leads to the "bended toe" condition, but they can also result when a toe or toes are too long and are forced into a cramped position when tight shoes are worn. They have also been known to be hereditary, and it is said that those with certain medical conditions, such as diabetes, are at increased risk for developing hammertoes as well. When aggravated, a corn or callus will build up on the toe, becoming inflamed and painful. With hammertoes, as with bunions, it's best to see a podiatrist or orthopedic doctor for evaluation and treatment as early as possible. He or she may recommend nonsurgical options such as prescriptive pads to shield the toe(s) from irritation. Over-the-counter pads are also available; however, skip those that are medicated as they often contain acid that can further the irritation. You should also avoid shoes with pointy toes, tight toe boxes, and high heels, which will push your foot against the front of the shoe and cause pain. Orthotics may be prescribed, as they can offer some relief as well as help shift the imbalance; they are also great foot savers for those with flat feet. In terms of less invasive procedures, your doctor can also administer corticosteroid injections to ease pain and relieve the inflammation without any downtime. Surgery, on the other hand, is a commitment, depending on the severity of your condition. Procedures such as arthroplasty can involve removing bone from the joint, while arthrodesis fuses the toe joint to straighten it. Finally, there are also surgical options that involve correcting the muscles and tendons to balance the joint. If your doctor recommends surgery, examine all options thoroughly, including your expected recovery time, so you can plan your life accordingly.

As for Yours Truly, I decided to stop buying shoes that only have room for four toes instead of five! I know the "last" (shoe form) and the designers/companies that work well for my feet, and I stick to them. I don't ever count on shoes stretching, nor do I bother trying to break them in. If they don't fit, I leave them at the store. In fact, I had a "closet confidential" conversation with my shoes recently and I told them, "You look great, but some of you will not be moving forward with me; many of you are too loose, some of you put the squeeze on me, and the rest of you don't earn your residency as all you do is just sit there without making a contribution because you don't play well with others, so you've got to go!"

Style Takes That Nail a Look

Shop Call

Do get yourself several pairs of long rubber gloves and a few "deli sheers" (you know, those transparent gloves the servers in the deli department wear), so whether you're cleaning the house or prepping food, your hands and nails are well protected. And while you're at it, why not treat yourself to an at-home hand-and-nail treatment with a body candle? It's like a paraffin experience, only better.

Show of Hands

Keeping your hands smooth and clear calls for targeted softeners and glow-getters. Here are some timeless picks:

- Clinique Even Better Dark Spot Correcting Hand Cream with SPF 15
- Deborah Lippmann Rich Girl Hand Cream with SPF 25
- Eucerin Advanced Repair Hand Creme
- Marini Luminate Hand Cream
- Nubian Heritage Coconut & Papaya Hand Cream

Shape Shifter

Nothing beats an almond-shape nail. Hands down, it flatters all and creates the illusion of long graceful fingers.

Playmates

Hot picks in nail hues abound, but some lines can be counted on year-round for what's "next." If your taste in lacquers ranges from the eclectic to the sublime, here are the lines with edge and wit to favor:

- Smith & Cult
- Nails Inc.
- Ciaté
- Butter London
- Dior
- Christian Louboutin
- Deborah Lippmann
- OPI
- Essie

Take Two

Looking for a nail twist? Why not try a matte-and-shiny combo? For instance, take a pale blue nail with a Bordeaux half-moon. Use a matte top coat on the pale blue and a shiny top coat on the half-moon. Other winning shade combos that translate:

- Black and white
- White and gold
- Silver and gold

Two Can Play That Game

When it comes to time-savers, there's nothing like having a combo mani-and-pedi experience, along with a playful color duet on tips and toes. At times I favor a nude hue on my fingernails and a deeper tone on my toes because the toes don't chip, and when lighter hues chip, they don't shout, "I need a manicure!" However, as we do with any accessory, there are times when we switch up and play with color on both. When I do, it's about a long-wearing gel formula that'll go the distance. So if you're in the mood for a duo that's très chic, book your appointment and spring for:

Nails	Toes
Orange	Red
Robin's egg blue	Bubblegum pink
Slate blue	Black cherry
Mint green	Lilac
Pastel pink	Pistachio
Powder blue	Pale pink

Say "Ah"

Close a day of high impact with a foot soak of Epsom salt and milk, followed by a self-massage using arnica oil or gel (chill in the fridge) to soothe and reduce muscle tension.

Shopping Cart

There's nothing like prime DIY picks that deliver pro peel results.

- Miss Spa Exfoliating Foot Booties, with glycolic acid
- Baby Foot (www.babyfoot.com), like a pro chemical peel for the feet
- NeoStrata Ultra Smoothing Lotion, with glycolic acid to gently exfoliate
- Amopé Pedi Perfect foot file, uses diamond crystals to smooth skin in minutes

Notes to Self...

Notes to Self...

5

Hair: Running the Show

Black women are the coif chameleons of the world. The journey to our many incarnations of style began in our earliest existence, when we created the most fascinating crowns of the ages to express our vision of our divine beauty. We gave birth to the rituals of washing, combing, and nourishing our hair with precious oils for hours in the motherland and, through this, the first protective hairstyles in history, along with a hair language all our own. Having been at the forefront of reporting on our journeys from the times when we couldn't wear braids and naturals to work and when advertisers homogenized our beauty by transforming us into carbon copies of other cultures, I know "the state of us." The beauty we celebrate surrounding our hair today and the fostering of what has truly become a more diverse narrative that speaks unapologetically to the power of our crown is in no way small, or a "just do you" moment, its quite symbolic of a revolution!

There was a time when the handful of products available to us could be memorized by a child because pioneer-owned hair care companies were fighting mainstream retailers for shelf space. We were the invisible women whose beauty wasn't depicted in ads. In fact, right through the early '00s, I found myself accompanying the *Essence* sales team on visits to beauty companies to help them understand the simple: you need to speak directly to us authentically through ads with visuals that resonate with us and with products developed for our distinct needs and styling desires. Beyond the magazine we had the Black church and beauty salons swelling our communities where we could share our hairstories, be inspired by style fellowship and care solutions, because we didn't have the global conversations we're having today on the internet that have changed the game. Though there have been improvements, things still aren't what they could be, and "ethnic hair care," as it's commonly referred to by retailers and mainstream companies, is still lacking, despite the fact that without our dollars their doors would be shuttered. And beyond the fact that we still have to manage skewed views of our various textures and distinctive hairstyles that spike debates and bans, we are woke and showing out! We are exploring all style options with purpose, making the journey back to natural with a passion that won't quit, and showing the world the full spectrum of possibilities as we redefine the way we are seen and heard. Freedom of choice aside, we have the most fragile hair on earth due to its natural curl pattern *and* given our instinctive desire to be our most creative selves, this calls not only for a style strategy but a new take on the age-old rituals of hair care.

66 **E**verybody's hair grows at the same rate regardless of ethnicity and texture. If you're not retaining your growth, you never got a real handle on hair care."

—Anthony Dickey, author, product innovator,
owner of Hair Rules Salon, NYC

Let's Talk Growth

Forget any notions that your hair doesn't grow. Unless it's impacted by stress, extreme dieting, endocrine function, hormonal disorders, scalp conditions, or any process that has permanently damaged your hair follicles (e.g., chemical burns, tension styling, scarring), nothing interrupts the flow. According to Dallas trichologist Rodney Barnett, our hair is always engaged in one of three cycles: growth, otherwise known as anagen; a rest or dormant stage known as catagen; and a shedding phase, telogen, where hair drops off and is replaced by new strands. In general, hair grows a half inch every month; however, the aging process does have an impact. "As we begin to get older, the growing cycle doesn't last as long," Barnett says, comparing it to the slowed cell turnover that also occurs as part of the aging process; however, it's what happens on the other side of that follicle that determines whether or not any amount of growth is retained. Experts cite popular styling practices as a common cause of hair breakage. "I'm seeing damage from women using the wrong products for their hair type due to myths and miseducation from growing up like 'Don't wash your hair for a month and it'll grow,' from YouTube channels full of mistaken information, from relaxers, which are the number one killer due to overlapping of the relaxer onto previously relaxed hair and the many misconceptions about them," celebrity stylist Amoy Pitters says, lamenting that all of this damage is "easily preventable." Certainly the misuse of relaxers has caused us a lot damage. "It's such a harsh chemical, even though it can work for those that favor it to loosen their natural curl pattern, but it's been abused for so long, and women of color have been programmed that it's the only way their hair is going to look nice," says celebrity stylist Tym Wallace. And we have abused relaxers by straightening out our entire curl pattern with the wrong strengths in our desire to be ultra-straight. "In navigating the myths and the mockeries surrounding your hair, there's a need to have some gatekeepers in place. For me, that's education," says hair authority Anthony Dickey, who's behind the style-setting looks worn by Jill Scott and Solange Knowles.

Every move you make has an impact on your hair. Don't test it!

Mikki-ism

Ahead of the Curve

There's no time like the present to prevent hair challenges by putting a plan in place that supports healthy hair from within and coupling that with well-suited styling practices. No matter how many luxurious hair products we use, nothing will result in the strong, healthy strands we desire if our diet is unhealthy. According to Dr. Ro, we must give ourselves more attention from an internal perspective. "This means getting those all-important B vitamins, especially biotin for healthy hair," she notes. In fact, Dr. Ro has a checklist that includes:

- Iron, which helps deliver oxygen to organs and cells, including our hair.

- Zinc, which supports hair growth (think pumpkin seeds, turkey, and lamb).

- Vitamin D, which supports healthy hair follicles (mushrooms, salmon, beef liver, whole unprocessed grains).

Style Codes

Don't try to reinvent the wheel yourself. Partner with a pro for your best takeaways, starting with the texture and condition of your hair for a treatment regimen that's conducive. "When it comes to getting the right information, you should invest the time to see a hairstylist for a consultation. This will in turn give you more agency over your hair at home," says Dickey. Truth is, we've been so used to shopping alongside professionals in barber and beauty supply stores because mass retailers failed us that we've become accustomed to analyzing our hair and treating it, but without professional knowledge, we can do a lot of damage. Celebrity stylists like Wallace, who keeps actress Taraji P. Henson tressed for success, urge us to remember that we shouldn't cut corners when it comes to our hair. "You don't diagnose or medicate yourself when it comes to your health, and you shouldn't diagnose your hair yourself," he emphatically states. The added value of a hair consultation is that the stylist will not only determine the condition of your hair, but will also indicate what your hair can and cannot take, as well as ascertain what you're able to execute and maintain in the style category in ways that aren't detrimental to your hair. According to Pitters, who emphasizes hair care at her tony NYC salon, Amoy Couture Hair, the value of partnering with a regular stylist should also be seen as a preventive measure. "When a client is well-informed on what to do, they don't come back into the salon with damaged hair," says the busy stylist, whose clients include actress Alfre Woodard and one of the most sought-after models in the world, Joan Smalls. Clearly, the best relationships are reciprocal, so do your due diligence and get the necessary information concerning your hair. When you work with an advised checklist of styling and conditioning aids, as well as the proper tools, you're supporting what's being done in the salon. Another smart move when having your consultation and subsequent hair appointments is to nail a coterie of your best style options and record the how-tos on video.

Protect and Serve

66 I t's not just about your hair looking good but making sure your hair is cared for."

—Kim Kimble, celebrity stylist

In the Trenches

When you get right down to it, for hair that's as dry and delicate as ours, hydration is essential. We can take nothing for granted as everything from the commonalties of everyday living, such as sleeping on cotton pillowcases, to combing and brushing, as well as how you style, has an impact on your hair. When you couple this with the rigors of maintaining a look, be it the frequent use of heated appliances, tension-driven styles, or such chemical processes as relaxers and permanent color, we can see why our hair, if not properly cared for, will succumb to damage. "I think a lot women run into trouble when they chase trends and fads, but the beauty of maintaining healthy hair lies in finding what works and sticking to it," says celebrity hairstylist Oscar James, whose expert care and styling techniques are favored by women in the spotlight like Vanessa Williams and Nicki Minaj. In Dickey's gospel of hair rules, "Your hair doesn't come with a care tag, but just like you wouldn't walk your cashmere sweater over to the washing machine, you have to make it your business to understand how to care for your hair." There's no secret when it comes to what will keep hair strong, supple, and healthy. It requires a loving care regimen based on the appropriate products at the appropriate time, and it all starts with the shampoo you use.

Try a Little Tenderness

Choosing the wrong shampoo is like picking up a stick of dynamite: the results can be explosive. "One of the biggest culprits of damage to kinkier curly textures are shampoos. They have made the hair industry trillions of dollars over the years, but for a long time they weren't historically made for women of color," says Dickey. High-sudsing shampoos—those that contain sodium lauryl sulfate and sodium laureth sulfate (also widely used in detergents)—will strip much-needed oils from your hair, cause it to tangle without mercy as they lift the cuticle of your hair, and ultimately lead to breakage. "You want to steer clear of detergent-based shampoos as detergent is for clothes, not your hair," Wallace adds. For dry, curly, color-treated, or chemically straightened hair, experts recommend the use of a sulfate-free shampoo (gentle, suds-free cleansing) to help retain moisture and elasticity as sulfates also make hair brittle and cause a dry, itchy scalp. Nonsudsing shampoos cleanse, balance, and refresh without stripping or depleting our hair of its natural oils with conditioning agents that gently lift product buildup and cleanse the scalp. What this means for curly and relaxed hair is that you can cleanse and detangle during the shampoo phase. Still, your salon professional is the best guide to how and when you should co-wash (incorporate the use of a cleansing conditioner) or use a conventional shampoo as part of your regimen. If you have scalp concerns, you should go a step further and also consult your dermatologist on the best shampoo to add to your product picks. In general, when shampooing, you always want to leave a little *slip* to the hair, as the pros say, as opposed to a squeaky-clean finish. Generalities aside, what constitutes an appropriate shampoo is affected by such factors as:

◉ How you wear your hair.

◉ If your hair is natural or relaxed.

◉ The condition of your hair and scalp.

◉ How often you shampoo.

◉ Your lifestyle.

This represents the kind of information essential to your discussions with your hair care professional and should ultimately influence your purchases.

Cleansing Agents

At a glance, here's a review of sulfate-free shampoo types for your checkout list:

- **Protein:** Cleanses and strengthens fragile hair, replenishes natural protein.
- **Conditioning/moisturizing:** Cleanses, coats, and protects the hair.
- **Co-wash:** Cleansing conditioner.
- **Clarifying:** Removes buildup from styling aids.
- **Dandruff:** Checks flaky scalps.
- **Color-treated:** Protects color from fading during the cleansing process.

Shopping Cart
- Hair Rules Daily Cleansing Cream
- Vernon Francois Curl Shampoo
- Creme of Nature Sulfate-Free Moisture & Shine Shampoo
- Kim Kimble Silk Treatment Shampoo
- Redken All Soft Shampoo
- Carol's Daughter Lisa's Hair Elixir Clarifying Sulfate-Free Shampoo
- L'Oréal EverPure Sulfate-Free Color Care System Moisture Shampoo

66 "Unfortunately, women are looking for miracles from their conditioner due to the damage caused by their shampoo. There's limited capability of what a conditioner can do if your shampoo is drying your hair out."

—Anthony Dickey

Take Charge

Today's conditioners are both change agents and maintenance guards for protecting your hair. On the appearance track, the right conditioner will detangle and keep your hair soft, shiny, and frizz-free. At a deeper level, you can expect intense hydration, revitalization, and fortified strands. There are distinct advantages to leave-ins, instant conditioners, and hair masks, and each has its purpose in the look and feel of your hair. "A leave-in conditioner acts as a barrier, similar to a moisturizer before makeup," says Dickey. I favor a leave-in that's used in the salon when my hair is wet to smooth and act as a heat protectant before blow-drying. Available in a variety of delivery forms, from sprays to lotions, there's a leave-in for every purpose. Instant conditioners are lightweight treatments used post shampoo to detangle and lubricate, and though they are rinsed away, they do smooth and impart light hydration. According to James, this is when you want to think like a pro and take this three-step approach: "One, make sure you comb the conditioner through as you want the hair to be just as tangle-free after you're done. Two, always use lukewarm water. And three, make sure you're not overrinsing the hair." Your hair mask, on the other hand, means serious business and, much like a facial, revitalizes and hydrates thirsty locks with such restructuring ingredients as hydrolyzed keratin, which strengthens hair by increasing its elasticity and moisture-binding capabilities. You'll benefit the most from this type of conditioning, so it's worth taking your stylist's advice if he or she determines it's time. If this is part of your advised at-home care regimen, be sure to not skip the process of adding heat, either with a hooded dryer or with a cap and a hot towel, as heat enhances the absorption of your conditioner.

Cut-Off Date

Having your ends trimmed every four to six weeks is part of a healthy care regimen. Think of it this way: as the most aged hair on your head, the ends have paid their dues, and now they must be snipped to prevent them from working their way up your strands and damaging the rest of your hair. Aside from the health of your hair, staying on top of this will shave styling time off your schedule as straggly ends always require more control. In between trims, buffer your ends with a little extra conditioner, especially when using heat appliances.

Fringe Benefits: Need-to-Know
Product Glossary

- **Dry shampoo:** Refreshes, neutralizes product buildup and oil, boosts volume.
- **Serum:** Smooths, adds shine, prevents frizz.
- **Gel:** Smooths, creates hold.
- **Hair butter:** Molds, sculpts, nourishes.
- **Liquid oil:** Renews, lubricates, nourishes, imparts shine.
- **Curl definer:** Intensifies curls, nourishes, defrizzes, heightens shine.
- **Wrap/setting lotion:** Adds body, provides a smooth set or wrap, prevents frizz.
- **Mousse:** Creates fullness, adds body, defines.
- **Hair cream:** Replenishes, hydrates, adds shine.

- **Holding spritz:** Imparts flexible control.
- **Light pomades:** Softens, lubricates, polishes.
- **Waxy pomades:** Provides medium hold, defines, adds shine.
- **Heat protectant:** Buffs against heat, improves straightening, resists humidity.
- **Sheen spray:** Adds shine, protects.
- **Straightening treatment:** Progressively straightens with each use, provides a barrier against humidity.

Hair tools aren't only accessories to great style—they're investment pieces. For the sake of your hair's health, don't skimp!

Mikki-ism

Tool Chest

- **Wide-tooth comb:** For detangling.
- **Blow-dryer:** A multitasker with (1) a diffuser to disperse air flow without disturbing hair's curl pattern, (2) a concentrator to smooth and straighten with direct air flow, and (3) a comb attachment to gently detangle hair and reduce frizz while drying.
- **Flexible setting rods (bendy rods):** For creating sleek spiral curls.
- **Tiny perm rods:** Great for tighter sets and enhancing texture.
- **Large hot rollers:** Perfect for adding volume.

- **Portable hooded dryer:** For effective drying, deep conditioning, and sets.
- **Ceramic flat iron:** Heats quickly and distributes heat evenly to straighten and smooth hair.
- **Tiny-barrel curling iron:** To add more definition to kinky/curly or relaxed hair.
- **Medium-barrel curling iron:** Versatile—creates voluptuous curls, smooths.
- **Large-barrel curling iron:** Creates big voluminous waves and lush curls.

Blowout: Mastering a Salon-Quality Blow-Dry at Home

I'm convinced there's an art to a great blowout, if for no other reason than the many hair bars across the country or the increasingly popular salons that now come to you. "Getting a silky finish is more about technique than anything—you have many wonderful tools, but it's all in the approach," James says. Investing the time in a 101 with your hairstylist is the best way to ensure you get the results you want at home. According to Pitters, "Your salon professional will make sure you have the right technique for your hair as well as the right blow-dryer, additional tools, and appropriate products." I've also learned that it helps if you have strong biceps, time (a minimum of twenty-five minutes, depending on the length of your hair), and patience. And trust me, a good cut or a healthy trim also helps as split ends, especially if your hair is natural, can be quite a challenge. When and where you blow-dry your hair is major, certainly: you do not want to execute this post shower in a humid bathroom as this will work against you. Now that the playing field is level, here's the straight shot to a fine finish:

A: Always shampoo and condition your hair first. "And be sure to use your conditioner liberally and be extra loving to your edges as they are most fragile," James advises.

B: Blot your hair until it's merely damp. Attempting to blow-dry sopping-wet hair is a setup for breakage with hair as fragile as ours because it increases the duration of both heat and tension needed to get the hair smooth and dry. Once you've toweled your hair, apply a leave-in conditioner. Some stylists prefer light sprays, others oils or a smoothing lotion. Keep the application light; whatever form you like, use less than you think you need unless you have natural hair. "The kinkier your hair texture is, the more you want to prep your hair before blowing it out by using a ton of leave-in conditioner and your favorite oils to coat and protect it while it's being stretched out," says Dickey.

D: Determine your objective. It's not about getting your hair too straight with the blow-dryer. "The flat iron does that," James says. You want to leave behind some body so the hair not only moves and looks salon-finished, but also looks polished and expensive. Section off your hair using a wide-tooth rubber comb to simplify the process, and avoid working on too large a section at a time or blow-drying randomly. If the objective is to blow your hair out in a specific style, part or section the hair accordingly.

N: Not all dryers are created equal, so it's important to choose the one that's most appropriate for your hair and styling needs and with the kind of technology (wattage capability) that gives you the best results in the shortest amount of time.

S: Start at the ends and work toward the roots if you're using a comb attachment. If you're using a brush, most experts prefer to see you use a paddle brush as opposed to a round metal brush as the metal heats up fast and can burn your hair; plus, the bristles are sharp and can tear your hair. Unfortunately, I know this to be all too true as when I used a round metal brush, I was popping strands by the minute and the broken flyaways weren't cute!

T: Take care not to hold the blow-dryer too close to your hair when using a brush. Hold it several inches from your hair and keep it moving. Blow-dry the hair one section at a time, pointing the concentrator of the dryer down the strands as you slowly pull the paddle brush down the length of your hair.

Straight Talk: Flat Irons 101

Growing up, I was a "press and curl" gal, and nothing straightened out my hair like a pressing comb! My mother could press hair like nobody's business, turning my fine kinky hair into corn silk every time. Did I hate the process? You better believe it. I never understood why I had to go through this torture every Saturday to worship the King on Sunday, but I must confess, I liked the results. Today flat irons are my manestay, but I don't subject my natural hair to the press. Instead, I test the latest and greatest out on my extensions. Like many of you, I like to look salon-fresh every day. Maybe that's why I've got a collection of flat irons in all sizes and such materials as ceramic and tourmaline, to straighten, smooth, and shape my hair. Though they're an important part of my style arsenal, I've learned to strike a balance when it comes to types and temperature settings, and the frequency with which I use them. Hair does have a glass ceiling, and I've learned the tough way, damaging my color-treated human-hair extensions in testing temps above 450 and plates that I should have passed on, so I know if you're not careful *and* informed, you can end up with dry, lifeless locks with a lot of breakage. Heat styling is enemy number one for relaxed and color-treated hair.

Flat irons are designed to be used on clean hair and, considering many of us don't shampoo our hair every day (with good reason), what does that tell us about frequent touch-ups during the week? Given that we have two to three styling/conditioning aids in our hair, flat-ironing over product buildup and pollution is a recipe for damage. But for those of us, Yours Truly included, who like to work a smooth, polished look or, alternatively, tousled waves, they're our MVPs, so using them while protecting the health of our hair calls for an approach that begins in the salon.

66 I f you're wrapping your hair properly, you shouldn't have to iron more than twice a week."
—Oscar James, celebrity hairstylist

When purchasing a flat iron, think quality, and be prepared to invest in the best iron for your hair as it'll save you money in the long run when you think about the alternative. When you get a quality straightener, you're guaranteed high performance. On the other hand, when you buy an inexpensive iron, you have to work harder as inexpensive plates often don't heat evenly. Don't be fooled by the price or the buzzwords used to market them; go for the kind of performance that only technology can deliver, and check the labels to be certain. A flat iron that features 100 percent ceramic plates (not nano-ceramic, which is a cheap composite) allows for even heat distribution and consistent results. A real plus in the retail market for us are ceramic irons that feature refillable tanks for adding hydrating ingredients like argan oil. I like to think of these revolutionary irons as the hair steamers of the day. The way I see it, I wouldn't press a silk dress with a dry iron. In fact, once you set the average iron on "silk," it indicates the need to add water. Salon pros like WE tv's *L.A. Hair* star Kim Kimble are taking matters into their own hands and putting technology to work. "I've been working on developing an argan-infused iron because they not only help protect the hair by buffering the heat, they add an unbeatable shine and the straightness lasts longer," Kimble says. Tourmaline irons also represent a great investment, and if you like exceptionally sleek results, this is your buy. Tourmaline, a crystal-born silicate, aids in the smoothing process by generating more moisture-locking ions than any other plate. It also seals in the hair's natural oils. Though a lot of people like titanium irons as they reach high temps, transfer heat more quickly than ceramic irons, and produce ultra-straight strands, I can tell you they will burn your hair if you're not careful, which is why I think they're best left in the hands of the pros.

Fine Lines

You shouldn't cut corners anywhere when it comes to your hair, so if you rely on a flat iron, please don't underestimate the importance of using an alcohol-free heat protectant as a buffer. Without this protective measure, you're asking for damage. Always iron your hair on the proper setting, and if you're not sure, get the advice of a salon professional and abide by it. Again, don't be tempted to go higher and put your hair at risk. Do take the time to section your hair off so you can work efficiently—take two or four sections, and clamp them in place with a plastic claw. Begin straightening your hair in small sections (one inch wide), and don't do more than two passes per section using fluid strokes, and keep it moving! You'll get smoother, even results by not ironing thick sections of hair. You'll also do far fewer passes, which means less heat and less damage control. Hairstylists like James prefer to start on the ends as they often don't get the proper attention. "I like to start there and give them one pass and then work from the roots down," he says, noting that a lot of today's styles feature a straighter end and "it's just a more modern look." Once you're done, add a pea-size amount of serum to the palm of your hands and run it through the hair to polish off your look, tame flyaways, and prevent any frizzing.

Wigs, Weaves, and Wherewithals

Due to changing attitudes and modern technology, wigs no longer have the negative connotation they used to have. For celebs and style chameleons alike, wigs represent a chic way to be a hair chameleon without taxing your hair. Whether it's a synthetic wig, a human-hair wonder, or an awe-inspiring lace front, today's wig looks nothing like the helmets of yesteryear. You can be as fabulous as you want to be in hue, length, texture, hairlines, and more, and all the while keep them guessing, "Is that her hair?" Not that this matters, because unless they're asking you who does your hair, it's none of their business! To me wigs are the real fascinators of the day as they allow you to express all of your mane takes and keep it moving in the style lane.

Before you shop, here are some elements of style to keep in mind:

- Select a wig based on your lifestyle and how often you intend to wear it.

- Ask yourself: Do I have a knack for styling? Time for maintenance? If so, a human-hair wig is your best pick; on an investment level, nothing beats a lace front wig. It doesn't get any more natural or versatile than this; however, be discerning about how often to play it because the daily use of the glue could cost you your hairline.

- If you want to have fun, are constantly on the go, and desire a quick, low-maintenance, affordable change whenever you're ready, then look for the quick chic of a synthetic wig that will retain its shape over time and is available in many style options.

Head Turners: Lace Front Wigs—Pros and Cons

Without question, a good lace front wig is a game changer, but like any style move that concerns our hair, there are pros and cons. According to celebrity hairstylist Ursula Stephen, a lace front wig is the highest-level wig in the category. "They're soft, lightweight, and very natural. However, a really good high-end human-hair full-lace wig is an investment that can cost between twenty-five hundred and three thousand dollars," says Stephen. Costs depend on whether the wig is hand-ventilated; whether it has a silk lace base that looks like a scalp on the whole wig or just at the front; and the length of the hair, as well as the color (e.g., a blond hue is more expensive as it takes more time to color the hair), but pros note that they last forever if properly taken care of. "And," adds Pitters, "when the lace matches our skin, it blends in seamlessly." Pitters favors lace front wigs with a silk base that allow you to experiment with partings, because they perfectly match your scalp and don't look heavy. Stephen says she's not seeing many of the high-end wigs because the market is flooded with inexpensive ones. "That means they're not going to be full-lace and therefore not breathable (read: not healthy for your hair and scalp), and aside from being heavy, they may be a bit tight or too big and potentially rub your hairline out," she notes. I've been blown away on the red carpet as well as in the studio watching the many incarnations and captivating personas wigs of this caliber provide. Perhaps that's the point, according to pros like celebrity hair mavens Amoy Pitters and Kim Kimble. "Celebs get them custom made, and going that route means you have to invest, but the advantage is the wigs are personalized in size and according to your skin color. That separates them from those that are sold in store by a man who knows nothing about hair," Pitters points out. Another advantage of investing in a customized wig as opposed to purchasing one at a beauty supply store is that you can get it repaired, and given the repeated wear, this should be important. "To have a wig done properly, have a stylist do it and know that custom is best," says Kimble, who's of the mind-set that lace front wigs were made for theatrical use and to adapt the hair in movies. "They're really a temporary option, as they weren't designed for everyday use because they require a lot of maintenance," says Kimble, who creates and styles them for films and television personalities.

Custom options aside, it's important to know what you're getting. Since there's no regulation of the content, a beauty supply store will say a wig is "100% human hair," but how can you know for sure? Though you can put heat on it, the question remains, *is* it 100 percent human hair? "It's impossible to regulate this—the market is wide-open," Pitters says, noting that anybody can sell hair under this pretense and make a profit. So, sis, I say look to your stylist or a reputable hair company and stick with it to be sure of getting the quality you deserve.

Beauty is the élan with which you live—don't compromise!

Mikki-ism

Everything we do has an emotional impact on our beauty. When you don't look great, you don't feel great. So anything that you choose to express your innate style—be it something as chic and simple as a lipstick or, in this case, a wig—is more than a notion because for us, beauty is always an emotional purchase. You especially want to be mindful of this before committing to a lace front, particularly if it's your first, and not only pour over your objectives but also keep in mind the integrity of your own hair. Certainly if hair loss is a concern, it's about not letting it disempower your self-esteem or compromise your style. In reality, you should have a coterie of options, and they don't all have to fall in the costly lace front category. Why not take the opportunity and work with a stylist and explore your best options across the category and think color, length, texture, and maintenance and have fun doing so? If hair loss isn't a concern, before you commit to a lace front, think about the role it will play in your life. Experts say when wigs are this fly, women can and do become dependent on them. "You become so used to wearing these wigs because you can sleep really well and wake up looking just as fabulous as the day before," says stylist Tym Wallace. Who wouldn't want that? However, it's like the old adage "When something is too good to be true, it usually is." "One of the cons of wearing a full-lace wig is it's addictive as it builds a dependency and takes away the idea of it being an accessory because you feel as if you can't go out without it," Stephen says. This kind of thinking sets the stage for damage. "When you wear a lace front wig this frequently, your hairline gets so thin that you *can't* go out without it," she pointedly adds. The message is loud and clear: everyday glam will cost you more than you anticipated if you work it overtime. "Lace front wigs are not to live in twenty-four hours. At that point, it's a weave, not a wig," says James, who feels the beauty of a wig lies in the styling options it provides. Keep in mind when you wear a wig of this nature every day, it's already taxing to your hairline, but if you're using tape or glue, there are added consequences. "Applying glue to the area every day can cause infection, and leaving the tape in causes it to pull out your hair and peel your skin," Pitters adds. So be diligent about removing the wig at night.

66 T ry a new cut, work a new color, but maintain the integrity of your hair."
—Oscar James

At the end of the day, it's always about protecting what lies beneath: your hair. For sure you need to moisturize before and after wearing a wig, and you'll definitely want to wear a wig cap or a protective stocking underneath. "Aside from getting your hair conditioned and braided, wearing a wig cap prevents friction on your hair," Pitters says.

66 Today, no one cares what people think. It's 'This is how I felt today and I'm proud of it!' I'm glad women are stepping out from hiding or being ashamed of wearing extensions."

—Carla Gentry Osorio, celebrity stylist

Weave Intel

I had my first experience with short-term extensions when graduating from the eighth grade. My mother had a human-hair fall made for me in the exact hues of my relaxed hair, complete with comb attachments to extend the length of my cascade curls. Come Sunday and birthdays, it was all about the possibilities with my newest accessory. Looking at it from this perspective at a young age was a healthy way to think about it. Ever the hairdresser, my mother emphasized the importance of taking care of my own hair first rather than putting the emphasis on the hairpiece. Though many years have passed and I've had a lot of style incarnations with extended options, this concept of taking care of my own hair sticks with me and is of the utmost importance to stylists today.

It's paramount that the technique and the style you choose don't hinder you from properly caring for your hair and scalp. You want to follow a care regimen that doesn't damage your hair or cause trauma to your scalp. This means making sure that your hair isn't braided too tight (this causes a form of hair loss known as traction alopecia, a direct result of tension on the hair follicle) and that too much hair isn't applied to areas where there isn't enough hair to support it, which also weakens strands and leads to breakage or permanent hair loss. Keep track of your appointments so that you don't wear weaves or extensions longer than eight to ten weeks. For those who are tempted to leave them in longer, know that you can very well incur hair damage, as well as "some type of bacteria at the scalp," Dickey warns. So take your cue from your stylist and make sure to have your extensions removed on time and have your hair shampooed, intensely conditioned, trimmed, and rebraided. In the meantime, remember a healthy scalp produces healthy hair, so don't skip your weekly shampoos and the opportunity to apply products that nourish and calm a dry and itchy scalp.

POWER POINT

More often than not we focus on texture, color, and style choices; however, stylists indicate there's so much more to be considered.

The Long View

Nowadays selecting the right hair involves such details as the origin of the hair and how it's been processed to how *versatile* the texture is as the question of longevity and versatility must be assessed. "I prefer hair that allows for versatility, mostly curly, so you can change the texture and wear it straight or curly. I also find virgin Indian hair is best," says Pitters, who's opened a hair boutique known as the Shop at Amoy Couture Hair, offering top-quality virgin Indian hair that's been hand sewn on a weft. Today there are so many types of hair on the market from various countries, and even then the origins are debatable, so it can be confusing. What it really comes down to is a question of quality, what works best for you and your lifestyle. With the going price for a professional sewn-in weave starting at approximately $1,200, I can tell you that you'll want to invest in the type of hair that will not only meet your needs and keep pace with your styling desires, but also hold up through repeated shampoos. "You also want to make the investment in great hair because you can use the hair over and over again for redos, touch-ups, so it's worth it," James advises. I've been disappointed by hair that's not as it was billed, so please make sure that the hair you choose can be put back in and that it can take color—even if you have to buy a sample to test it—because custom color is part of what turns a look from great to amazing! Color aside, nothing can be more disappointing than investing in hair that doesn't hold up and as a result begins to look dull, fake, and rough, and tangles or frizzes throughout the day. I know that despite your best efforts, the treatment products and megawatt tools, nothing can improve the look and behavior characteristics of poor-quality hair, so think twice before you spring for that bundle that only costs $20 or $30 as it's most likely not 100 percent human hair. It's like tossing money out the window and you wouldn't do that, so it's best to purchase hair through your stylist or a reputable resource.

Feeling Haute

If you're a sister who likes to explore options in style, color, length, and/ or texture, human-hair extensions offer the experience as well as the freedom* minus the long-term commitment, let alone the avoidance of stressing your own hair. "Hair extensions are more of an accessory now. It's no longer the stigma of 'I have a weave so that means I don't have any hair,'" says celebrity hairstylist Carla Gentry Osorio. Many celebrities and models alike take this route to work their style and color options as well as to save their own hair from the stress of double processing, lots of heat, and the many styling demands that come with being on duty in the public eye, which can be damaging to their hair as well. Hairstylist Tym Wallace, who's behind the fresh looks worn by such A-list sisters as Kelly Rowland and Brandy, says that he's always focused on the integrity of his clients' own hair and admires those celebs who have the confidence to do what's best for their hair. "A celebrity will say, 'Let's cut it off if it's damaged, let's start over, let's braid it up,' so that courage of not being afraid to get rid of dead hair and don a wig or put in a weave is a smart move," Wallace says. Now there's not a day that goes by where you and I feel we don't have to look our best, so the same thinking of not taxing our hair or doing what we have to do so we can be as fierce as we want to be makes sense. What it comes down to is determining your look(s), the costs involved, and how much time you have to devote to maintenance. "Maybe you don't have a lot of time in the morning and you want to get up and go, so you might choose hair that has a slight wave texture so you don't have to straighten it," Stephen says. For stylists like Oscar James, it all starts with a picture. "I like working with a visual so nothing gets lost in translation; then it's about lifestyle, a person's wardrobe, and how savvy they are when it comes to styling their hair," he says. Perhaps you'll want to work your own hair in at the hairline (known as a leave-out) as part of the look. "I'm always thinking about the end results, so I check out the hairline to determine if we're going to do a closure [a small hairpiece that's sewn in to cover the crown that allows one to create the illusion of a part] or a leave-out," says Stephen. Keep in mind that if you choose to do a leave-out, pampering your edges is a must because the hair will go through a little more when styling. What's also key here is choosing a texture that complements your own. So it's really a question of weighing your options against your lifestyle and what's required to maintain the look you have in mind, as well as placing yourself in the hands of an expert stylist with a great resource for quality extensions and style know-how.

> 66 Extensions should make your life easier and the styles you choose effortless."
> —Ursula Stephen, celebrity hairstylist

Style Works

Whether you want to work a fierce fro, sexy spirals, free-flowing twists, fierce braids, perhaps a fresh pixie or an elongated bob, great textures abound. Some styles translate well with human-hair extensions, and some work better using synthetic hair due to its sturdiness.

Human-hair extensions are always going to be softer, more compatible with your own hair, and offer you greater versatility; however, they do require more maintenance. Though durable, synthetic hair is harder on our natural hair because it can both cut the hair and dry it out. Many stylists recommend that you minimize the amount of time you leave synthetic extensions in because of these characteristics, advising removal after a four- to six-week period, followed by deep conditioning of your natural hair. Once you've decided on your look, texture, and type of hair, you'll want to work the freshest dos. This is where products, tools, and techniques enter in. When I went for a bang and an elongated bob, I had to learn how to blow-dry my hair with a brush. As previously indicated, I tried a round brush, which not only made me feel like I had two left hands, but when I finally got it right, I realized that though the body was great, the breakage was a problem. When I switched to a wooden paddle brush, it was easy-breezy. I also went through a serious array of flat irons to find those that worked best for my extensions and found that tools from companies like Kimble Hair Care, BaByliss, and Bellezza work best. Let's say you're preparing to wear a twisted bob: for you that might mean purchasing hair butter and knowing how to twist and release your hair. "It all depends on the texture. If it's waved, you'll need a curling wand; if it's curly, a curling iron to wrap the curls around when it's necessary to reinforce the texture or define the overall shape; straight and sleek, a flat iron and wrapping properly at night," James says. All of these choices indicate that your style and maintenance moves should be well thought out.

Extensions should be fabulous, fun, and liberating, yes— however, like any other beauty move, you get out of it what you put into it. That means maintenance, maintenance, maintenance!

Mikki-ism

Well Tressed

"The worst thing that can be said is 'Your weave looks great.' They should be saying, 'OMG, your hair looks great,'" says Stephen, for whom it's always about the look and the feel of the hair. Certainly there's no shame in wearing extensions, but at the same time, you still want to slay by taking care of them. There have been many late nights when all I wanted to do was fall in bed and call it a day, but because I want to keep my investment in the best of care, I always take the time to wrap my hair properly and put on a silky scarf to prevent dryness. If you've chosen to wear extensions, then you've also happily chosen the upkeep that goes along with doing so in order to look well tressed. Keeping your extensions polished and in perfect condition while making coif changes calls for a lot of TLC and a consistent care regimen to protect your hair. Think hydration, and cleanse your hair weekly with a moisturizing shampoo that's both paraben- and sulfate-free so you can protect your extensions from becoming dry and brittle, especially if your extensions are colored as products with sulfate will strip your color. To treat and smooth, always follow with an instant conditioner and make sure to gently comb your hair out from the *ends* to the base and rinse with luke-warm water. Pay attention to your hair, as there will be those times when you'll need to deep condition. Pitters says, "Practices like the repeated use of a flat iron can cause the cuticle to become rough, and using a deep conditioner will seal it and restore smoothness." If you wear a sleek look, be sure to steer clear of oily products to avoid weighing down the hair and causing it to become limp and lose its body. "Oily products as well as silicone-based products act like a coating on top of the hair, and because they don't penetrate, you get a buildup," Pitters notes. So be ingredient savvy when flying solo by checking labels. Kimble advises clients at her West Hollywood salon, Kimble Hair Studio, to use the same care and styling aids the pros use as they are constantly educating themselves on ingredients and treatments. It's no wonder she and other stylists like Amoy Pitters, Anthony Dickey, and London-based Vernon Francois (go-to stylist for such celebs as Lupita Nyong'o, Ruth Negga, Cynthia Erivo, and others) have also created their own lines, not only to give women salon-quality results at home regardless of whether or not they wear extensions but to yield what they're looking for in terms of product performance overall.

Purchasing a good hooded dryer is also an important part of car-ing for your hair as you must be sure to dry your hair thoroughly and this takes time, especially if your extensions are sewn onto a pre-braided cap. Neither a blow-dryer (though it allows you to achieve faster, sleeker results) nor a diffuser (which will dry curly textures, while leaving them intact) effectively dries the base of your weave and the blow-dryer places additional stress on both the extensions and your own hair.

So Illuminating

Certainly you'll want to aim for those styling aids that will keep your look healthy and lustrous, and that translates into avoiding any styling aids containing alcohol, which is drying. Depending on your texture/style, you may need a heat protectant, an antifrizz serum, a curl definer, or a dry shampoo. I especially rely on dry shampoo to keep my bangs fresh as they're the next best thing to hitting a blow-dry bar as they renew, check oil, and put an airy bounce back into slack strands. As a bang devotee, I know they can be compromised by everything from the natural oils on my forehead to the elements, product buildup, and heat damage. To keep them from separating or, worse, wilting on me, Pitters, who I see on the regular, taught me how to spray dry shampoo onto a brush and pull it through my bangs from underneath, and the gratification is instant. I also use Velcro rollers to add shape and volume while I'm doing my makeup (better than repeated use of a flat iron). For a glossy finish, I follow the pros and keep it light. "I like serums and a good spray sheen as they give a great weightless gloss to the hair," James says. Color-warming hues or highlights also up the glow factor.

Night Moves

To keep your look salon fresh and prevent matting, be sure to wrap your hair at night with a silky scarf or a satin bonnet. If you wear braids, a stocking cap or a do-wrap (no rags for the Queen!) will keep your hair in place and frizz-free. If you wear soft waves or curls, pin-curl your hair and wear a satin bonnet. Remember, your nighttime objective is to protect your hair, so it's important to avoid moisture-zapping cotton scarves and pillowcases.

Curl Cues: Transitioning from Relaxed to Natural

Calling It Quits

How does it feel to be a beauty CEO? For those of us who have gone natural and by doing so started a movement that changed the hair care industry and retail offerings, it feels amazing! Until recently, we were relegated to a few pitiful shelves in store with very little diversity in the products that were offered to us, and that off-putting reality caused our salon owners and indie hair care companies to take matters into their own hands by creating products for a new generation of natural hair Queens. It made retailers sit up and take notice and carry more diverse products from existing hair care companies that previously had difficulty getting an array of picks in this category in store as well. It also caused hair care companies to invest in the kind of technology that would produce products better suited to our natural curl pattern and how we like to style. But the big by-product of our determination to raise the bar and celebrate our beauty was the number of us who, in making the transition, discovered just how versatile our natural textures are. One of the many things I love about the natural hair movement, as someone who's watched our journey for years, is this: gone is the notion that you can't work out! Truth is a lot of us were relegated to hairstyles our entire lives that kept us away from the gym and, in particular, water. Think about it: How many times have you gone to the spa and wanted a Vichy shower or desired to dive off a boat in the Caribbean? But now you can take your natural hair into any experience and not sweat it! "Who knew your hair wanted a wash-and-go style," says Dickey. Thanks to the movement, this is a new conversation for women of color.

It also signaled just how versatile our natural textures are. For stylists like Dickey of NYC's Hair Rules Salon, which specializes in natural hair, it caused women to begin to look at their natural textures in a different light. "So it not only helped to usher in the retail landscape of products that once weren't available for us, but an internet community full of empowering stories that said our hair texture is not bad, this is the way God made me, my natural hair is really beautiful," says Dickey. The movement not only called for new products and style options, but also, for those embracing their natural hair for the first time since childhood, it began a journey that calls for transitional practices to preserve our hair. Making the transition can be a traumatic move if not done with knowledge, care, and a commitment to restful styles that are long on looks and short on manipulation. To successfully accomplish this while retaining your new growth requires a game plan that coddles hair, particularly where the two textures meet, and allows you to keep your style quotient intact during the process.

Twists and Turns

Your first determination in the journey back to natural is to decide whether it will be a gradual process or if you'll liberate yourself immediately by making what stylists call "the big chop." I've seen many sisters take the former approach and discover a side of themselves they never knew existed as they learn about products that enhance their textures and allow them to wear diverse looks. For years, we've believed our natural hair was limiting and that relaxed textures gave us more options. Not so! Take, for example, actress Lupita Nyong'o and her many style takes in the public eye. Whether it's through partings, edgy shapes, or even the way her hairstylist Vernon Francois works height and volume, it's one sensational look after another. For you that might mean growing out an inch or so of your natural hair and cutting off your relaxed hair and exploring coils or extensions that mimic your texture and offer more styling options.

Curl Tactics

If you decide to retain your length and not cut your hair, you'll want to either put a stationary style in place or a style that doesn't cause a lot of manipulation as the point where your new growth and relaxed hair meet is extremely vulnerable. "If your natural hair has a very tight curl pattern, you're going to get breakage," says the busy bicoastal stylist Carla Gentry Osorio, who's behind the camera-ready looks of Kerry Washington and Shonda Rhimes. Begin by placing the care and styling of your hair in the hands of a professional stylist to strategize your best regimen of trims, products, and healthy style tips. This is where your stylist can recommend style options that will last from shampoo to shampoo and moisture-conscious products to lubricate and minimize damage. The transition phase represents a time to coddle your hair and get to know it better as it grows out. According to Dickey, who transitioned BET CEO Debra Lee into her ultrachic crop, this reacquaintance allows you to understand what your hair does and what you need to do to care for it. "Our biggest message for women coming in and wanting to investigate their natural hair or are transitioning is that of helping them understand that there's a whole grading system based on texture," Dickey says. Textures are graded in the salon on grafts that define natural curl patterns from #2 wavy to #4 kinky. Essentially, most Black women have #3 curly or #4 kinky hair, and yes, you can possess more than one texture. "You can do anything to your hair, but the grading system helps you understand which products and care practices will work best for your texture. Then you can say, this is what my hair does, here's what I need to do to care for it," Dickey says. When going natural, it's about understanding the two dominant textures, how to care for your hair overall, and what styling techniques are best as you journey from where you are to where you want to be.

Damage Control

One of the biggest culprits in damaging curly and kinky textures are shampoos, so here again sulfate-free shampoos are a must to avoid stripping your hair and to keep it soft and pliant. There's limited capability of what a conditioner can do if your shampoo is drying your hair out. These nonsudsing shampoos also allow you to detangle while washing your hair. Deep conditioning every week is also critical to your regimen, and this is where you want to be sure to distribute hair-nourishing treats from root to ends. The tighter your natural curl pattern, the more naturally dry your hair is and the more prone it is to tangle and break, so it's about keeping your hair infused with moisture through leave-in conditioners and your favorite fatty oils. Dickey advocates essential oils. "If you cleanse with something that's moisturizing, then there's no need to go in with heavy grease or waxes that compound the problem," he adds.

Style Forward

In an era of YouTube tutorials, visiting a professional stylist who can help you understand your specific texture and how it will respond to products and style techniques is your best bet. "You want clients to get to a point where they're enjoying their hair and you're enjoying doing their hair," says Osorio, of Manhattan salon Styles Beauty Lounge, who sees these amateur tutorials inflict carnage that she feels compromise the integrity of the hair. There's nothing more disappointing than going through a tutorial and not getting the results. For example, if you've got two inches of new growth and your natural hair texture is a #4 and the rest of your hair is still relaxed, a stylist will know what products and techniques will enable you to get a look that mimics your desire for Tracee Ellis Ross's sensuous fluffy curls. A YouTube tutorial will not. Professionals also can inform you how many days you can expect to get out of certain style techniques. Most stylists recommend "protective styling" during the transition phase as styles in this category are either stationary or require less manipulation and last longer. "I definitely recommend braiding your hair or doing a weave as it's easier to grow your hair out that way," says Kimble. For certain, pretreating with hydrating conditioners before you put your hair away for any length of time—and being mindful of good scalp care by using essential oils with therapeutic properties (tea tree oil, sage, basil) that nurture as well as check any itching—is necessary. Restful sets using perm rods or flexi rods are also great options as they not only allow you to achieve a consistent curl but also camouflage the area where the textures meet. Styles like this can be finger-combed into place, lessening your chances of breakage, and they last from week to week. "So use what's available to you to style and keep in mind that time is a healer and how you think about the new hair coming in today is much different than eight months from now when you've got several more inches and you've been living with it," Dickey notes. And don't get frustrated! Fall in love with the process of discovery. Today's salons offer an array of styles, such as textured bobs, fros, coils, knots, braids, locks, and more, with or without extension support (matching textures now is a cinch), so don't think you have to grin and bear the transition or sport a teeny natural during the growth period—or for that matter become formulaic and lose your passion for change.

Hair Color: Setting the Tone

Rules of Engagement
Hair color is the force behind some of the boldest looks going, from the red carpet to the runways that are the streets of the world. We are living in an age of possibilities, and insta-glam takes with hair color is the "it" move in beauty. There's not one among us who will settle for drab hair, so even those who haven't committed to color will spring for a gloss to put texture and shine in the spotlight. Celebrities and trendsetting beauties favor statement-making hues, and whether you're a color chameleon like Rihanna, put a vivid stake in the ground like

Faith Evans, or work shimmering highlights around the face like Ciara, color allows for self-expression like nothing else in the beauty realm. It also allows you to play it rich and elegant with subtle strokes of color that add dimension, emphasize a cut, highlight a technique like braids or twists, or give new life to silver strands. Newer techniques also allow for blurred lines that obscure the transition between roots and ends, making regrowth less obvious and multiple tones more organic. "It's all about dimension—once you create that, the color is modern and more interesting," says James, who works with style mavens Halle Berry and Tyra Banks, whose looks consistently feature gradations of color. One of James's standbys is his three-color rule: dark under the bottom, light around the face to give a little pop, and darker roots, a strategy that he also applies to human-hair wigs, which makes them look so natural on the red carpet. If you're considering color, especially for the first time, or if you're looking to make a change, it's really important to see a colorist who understands how to achieve results without compromising the integrity of your hair. "You want to look at what can harm your hair—chemicals, color, extensions—and stay ahead of the game by seeing a professional," says the in-demand stylist and educator Kim Kimble. Working out your options with a professional colorist will help you determine your best move based on how often you're able to visit the salon for touch-ups, your lifestyle habits (e.g., whether you're a swimmer or exercise or travel frequently), costs associated with the process, both to your hair as well as your wallet, and other variables that can impact how long it will last.

66 **Y**ou want to splurge on color and maintenance because you're worth it!"

—Oscar James

Try a Little Tenderness

As long as we go to great lengths to style, we must also work the necessary maintenance to keep our locks in prime condition. Because our hair is naturally drier, any chemical process must be accompanied by lots of hydration in hair care and style support products. Remember, though, our hair is strongest in its virgin state; any color process beyond a temporary rinse can be drying. If you have relaxed hair, you'll want to steer clear of permanent color to prevent damage. If you want a color change that requires lightening or bleaching the hair, it's best to work with human-hair clip-on pieces to avoid double processing your hair. Kimble, who created Beyoncé's gilded look for *Lemonade*, feels so strongly about the risk of breakage with chemically treated hair that she determines who she will and will not color in the interest of their hair. "There are so many clients who want what I give my celebrity clients, but when you have over twenty-seven years of experience, you know what's not going to work or isn't in the best interest of the client because they won't be able to maintain it," Kimble says. In truth, the care of your hair lies more in your hands than it does those of your hairdresser, so at home you'll want to be diligent about staying on course from shampoo to shampoo. That means always using sulfate-free shampoos (sulfates strip moisture *and* color) and investing the time needed for a deep conditioner formulated for color-treated hair. It's about using those product picks geared to protect your color from fading. This is your time to baby your hair, so consider purchasing a hooded dryer and plastic caps for weekly treatments. Nourishing leave-in conditioners and alcohol-free styling aids should be incorporated into your regimen as well. If you have permanent color, keep heat styling to a minimum, and always use a heat protectant. If your hair is natural, hair color will cause it to be more porous, so it's of the utmost importance to use products that help seal the cuticle. Because of this your hair will absorb leave-in conditioners more quickly, so the use of light oils to help lubricate the hair and maintain softness will be key. Locks can take much longer to absorb color than virgin hair at the roots, and often calls for additional product; therefore it's best to have them colored, at least initially, by a professional. A pro will also take into account the age of your locks and be able to determine how often it's wise to color them to prevent breakage.

Personalizing Your Look at Home: Know Your Stuff

Honing your look at home calls for knowledge about color offerings, what's necessary to achieve the results you desire, and diligent care, all of which should be guided by your salon professional. "People buy color, and it's not always the formula that should be used, so you should always have your hair assessed by a professional first, and if they say, 'I don't think your hair can take the color,' listen to them," Osorio says. Once you have the green light, you'll really want to avoid a bottle color look by purchasing a formula that delivers a salon-worthy finish in its distinction and subtle nuances, so don't hesitate to ask your professional for guidance. Before you proceed to color, always patch test the product on your skin, to determine any sensitivity, as well as on a few strands to see if you like the results. Now here's a final primer on what and what not to do:

- Always follow instructions to the letter.

- Never apply color if your scalp is irritated.

- Deep condition hair in the weeks leading up to coloring and consistently thereafter.

- Always apply color to clean hair only, making sure to cover hair thoroughly from roots to ends for an even tone.

- Color takes best on healthy hair; if hair is damaged or breaking, see a professional for restructuring conditioners and, when appropriate, professional color.

⦿ Always wait at least two weeks between relaxer application and color.

Defining Color

Taking Stock, Making Note: Your Glossary at a Glance . . .

- **Rinse:** Does not penetrate, coats only the strands of the hair, enriches existing color, lasts approximately three to four shampoos; safe for relaxed hair, ammonia- and peroxide-free.
- **Semipermanent color:** Deposits color, lasts six to eight shampoos; gentler than permanent color, but still constitutes a double process when applied to relaxed hair.
- **Demi-permanent color:** Penetrates the hair shaft, contains a small amount of peroxide but doesn't lift, imparts some color, enhances natural color and covers gray, great for color-correcting in the hands of a professional, lasts up to twenty-four shampoos.
- **Permanent color:** Incorporates peroxide and ammonia to lift existing color and provide a permanent change; does not wash out but can fade; requires touch-ups for new growth depending on the application technique.
- **Conditioning color:** Imparts conditioning properties onto the hair and coats it during the color process, lasts four to six weeks; safe for relaxed hair.
- **Bleach:** Permanently removes natural pigment; used to highlight, lift color; taxes hair the most.

Hello, Sunshine!

Working super healthy hair with lots of shine calls for lots of hydration and brilliance-boosting shampoos, moisturizing hair masks, and shine serums as opposed to oily aerosol sprays that create buildup. What casts your radiance into next-level territory are color-warming hues (think rich bronzes, cola browns, and reds) and sun-kissed highlights (golds and ambers). Whether you chose a bottled bestie or colored clip-ons, you're just a step away from enhancing your hair's glow factor.

Losing Out Loud

Our hair is our crowning glory, and nothing threatens the crown like hair loss. The inexperienced might say, "It's only hair," but unless you've stood in the shoes of a woman who's losing her hair, you can't possibly understand why hair loss is a brutal and unfair challenge. It doesn't matter what age you are, what you do for a living, whether you're married or single, in school or commanding the C-suite, hair loss is an equalizer that can threaten the self-esteem of the best of us. Hair loss among Black women is reaching epidemic proportions, and while we have many visual options to deal with it, there's very little to address the looming stress within. It's about more than a great hairstyle; when you lose your hair, there's a complexity of emotions that rise to the surface and cause you to feel everything from dismay to guilt and back. "Well-meaners" will offer home remedies and chalk your loss up to your styling practices; they'll urge you to take this hair vitamin or try that hair food, but the best advice anyone can share is to recommend you to one of the following: a dermatologist who specializes in hair loss, a trichologist (hair and scalp specialist) for an examination, or a hair restoration physician.

According to the International Society of Hair Restoration Surgery, nearly thirty million women in the United States are losing their hair. Causes range from aggressive styling techniques to medications and internal disorders (see "Hair Loss Exposed," page 226, for causes). No matter the cause, this is the time to empower yourself by taking the necessary steps to get to the root of the problem for a solution at first sign. "Women have a tendency to go into denial, and rather than having these concerns diagnosed, they camouflage them by changing their hairstyle," says trichologist Rodney Barnett who regards hair loss as a warning sign. In fact, denial is said to be the reason hair loss goes on for years. The challenge that Barnett and others are seeing is that oftentimes women's hair loss is not addressed until we've lost about 40 percent of our hair. It doesn't help that companies are marketing all kinds of topical hair dressings and "miracles in a bottle" claiming to regrow our hair, but I need you to put your money away until you see a hair care professional who can refer you to a board-certified expert. As we look at what's taking place, many of us are losing our hair to one of the several types of alopecia that are affecting African American women the hardest. Here's what we can control and what we can't.

> " We now have an edges epidemic, from all the pulling and tightening. A lot of my clients have switched to wigs as opposed to weaves because they realize the tension isn't good."
>
> —Oscar James

Traction Alopecia

Traction alopecia, affecting the hairline, temples, and behind the ears, is the leading form of hair loss among us. Look, there's no sugarcoating this: it's caused by tension styling (weaves, braids, twists, tight dos) and the improper application of wigs. Wearing your hair in any technique that puts tension on your scalp or that results in red bumps, pus bumps, or flaking can damage hair follicles and cause scarring. "There is no coming back from tension alopecia as once the follicle comes out at the root, the hair isn't coming back," Kimble says. So it's best to get out in front of it with restful styling and game-changing treatments. Platelet-rich plasma (PRP) injections is one such treatment proven to be effective at the first sign of thinning. "Platelets that circulate in our blood contain powerful internal growth factors (IGF)," says Dr. Benjamin C. Paul, renowned hair restoration physician at HairCareMD in New York City, who's a proponent of PRP. When administering this procedure, a physician draws a small amount of blood from a patient, isolates the IGF using a centrifuge, and combines them with specific medicines to concentrate the anti-inflammatory components of the blood. This PRP is then gently and painlessly injected into the areas of the scalp affected by hair loss. The process takes thirty minutes and is repeated anywhere from once a month for three to six months to three times every six to eight weeks, followed by once every six months thereafter for maintenance. This A-list procedure minimizes thinning, causes new growth to be thicker in diameter, and many women begin to see a difference after two to three treatments.

No one could have told me that my signature look for years, pulling my hair back in a chignon, would contribute to losing my hairline, but it did and what a blow. At the recommendation of my longtime hairstylist Amoy Pitters, I paid a visit to Dr. Paul, who diagnosed my hair loss as Frontal Fibrosing Alopecia (FFA). Its characteristics, primarily a band of hair loss on the front and sides of the scalp, are much like traction alopecia but that's where the similarities end. FFA is slowly progressive and can cause one to experience loss of one's eyebrows as well, which I did. "The exact underlying cause of FFA is unknown but it is thought to be an autoimmune condition in which a person's immune system mistakenly attacks the hair follicles," he explained. Scientists also suspect that there may be a hormonal component since the condition most commonly affects postmenopausal women over age fifty. There is currently no cure for FFA; however, treatment with certain types of medications may stop or slow hair loss in some cases. Treatment often involves using anti-inflammatory medications or ointments, such as corticosteroids, tetracyclines, or hydroxychloroquine (brand name Plaquenil), to reduce inflammation and suppress the body's immune system. Medications that block the production of the male hormone 5-alpha reductase (finasteride) have been reported to stop further hair loss in some women. "In my experience, the combination of injectable steroids and PRP are effective at treating FFA, and I alternate these procedures monthly until quiescence of the FFA," Paul adds. Depending on the amount of hair loss, transplantation surgery, where hair from the back of the head (known as the donor site) is transferred to the area of loss, is also an option. Modern techniques focus on restoring the hairline and reinforcing density by transplanting larger numbers of hair grafts, which in turn reduce the number of procedures needed to achieve results. Transplanted hairs will continue to grow for life and maintain their natural characteristics in color and texture. Due to the length of time I'd waited, the area was deemed too large to address with transplantation, so Pitters created a look for me based on bangs and soft layers with extensions. But again, the real win is early diagnosis.

Androgenetic Alopecia

According to Barnett, who treats hair and scalp conditions at his facility in Dallas, twenty-one million African American women suffer from androgenetic alopecia (genetic thinning) alone. Unlike other types of alopecia, where something has been done to provoke them, with androgenetic alopecia, also referred to as "female pattern baldness," there's nothing that you've done to contribute to it; it's just a predisposition you inherited. It's worth noting, though, that if you wear locks or braids and have been diagnosed with androgenetic thinning, this will lead to traction alopecia if not considered, so you don't want to put tension and stress on your hairline or, in the case of extensions, add too much hair to this area. You'll want to inform your hairstylist of this diagnosis so modifications in chemical services and styling techniques can be made in the best interest of your hair. It might be something as simple as clip-on hair pieces, which represent a modern and temporary option, while you're under a doctor's care. Treatments like minoxidil (Rogaine) and laser therapy to stimulate cell growth represent noninvasive solutions; some medical professionals may also include prescriptive medications and possibly hormone therapy. Hair-restoration surgery may also be an alternative, but because thinning can occur on the donor areas such as the sides and back of the head, this can be problematic. In the meantime, don't be hard on yourself; work with a stylist to make those style discoveries that bring you joy and keep it moving.

Alopecia Areata

When the immune system specifically attacks your hair follicles, resulting in smooth, round patches of hair loss, this is known as alopecia areata. In most cases, hair grows back, but in rare cases it progresses to alopecia areata totalis, where all the hair is lost on the scalp, or alopecia areata universalis, complete loss of hair on your scalp as well as elsewhere on your body. Here again, experts don't know why the immune system attacks the follicles, though there are associated conditions, among them thyroid disease, collagen vascular diseases, and chronic stress; hair loss isn't permanent unless you have an autoimmune disease. This form of alopecia is diagnosed by a hair analysis as well as through blood tests to check your thyroid and your overall internal health to determine what's oppressing your immune system. Treatment therapies include corticosteroid injections or cream applied to the scalp along with minoxidil. Wigs and hair pieces on a light base can be worn to keep your style in check, but weaves and braids should be ruled out as they may cause permanent hair loss. You will feel most empowered by getting the jump on this through diagnosis, treatment, and style choices that don't compromise the way you like to look.

Central Centrifugal Cicatricial Alopecia

This form of alopecia begins at the center of the scalp and extends outward, scarring hair follicles as it slowly progresses. It is the most common form of scarring hair loss seen in Black women. Though the causes can be multiple, they are often associated with viral, bacterial, or fungal infections. Early diagnosis, which involves a scalp biopsy, is critical to prevent further progression and extensive, permanent hair loss. Treatment includes anti-inflammatory steroids, antibiotics, and immune suppressants. In the meantime, experts look to scalp care as a preventive measure. "It's a big myth that African American women can't shampoo their hair on a weekly basis, and the danger in this belief is that the scalp sweats and toxins are left to surround your hair follicles," Barnett indicates. This buildup, when not addressed, can cause inflammation, also known as folliculitis. So if you work out frequently or have extreme hot flashes, how often you shampoo is going to be different from someone who doesn't. For Kimble, who finds herself referring clients to dermatologists or hair-replacement specialists for surgery, prevention is always top of mind. "Bacteria in your hair can cause hair loss, so practices like taking your extensions down and making sure your hair and scalp are cleansed properly is a must," she cautions. That also means going the extra mile when you shampoo at home by making sure your extension tracks are completely dry because leaving them wet or damp can also lead to a bacterial breeding ground. It also means you must take care when wearing wigs because wigs raise the temperature of the scalp and also trap moisture, which is why you don't want to live in a wig round the clock. When all is said and done, one thing is certain: when you've done your best for the health of your hair and scalp, you have to remember you are not your hair, and however you work your crown, looking fly is within your power.

Hair Loss Exposed

Reasons for hair loss vary, but here's a list of common causes:

- Repeated and frequent chemical processing
- Tension styling
- Aging/menopause
- Heredity
- Medications (statins, blood pressure drugs, antidepressants, Accutane)
- Hormonal imbalances
- Thyroid conditions
- Chronic stress
- Anemia
- Extreme diets
- Endocrine disorders
- Vitamin deficiencies
- Autoimmune conditions

To find a dermatologist who specializes in hair disorders, visit the American Academy of Dermatology website at www.aad.org and click "Find a Dermatologist"; then enter your zip code and under "Specialty" tap "Hair Disorders."

Notes to Self...

Notes to Self...

6

Style: Make a Statement

Burberry had an advertising slogan that spoke so succinctly of its brand that said: "Wherever you experience Burberry, it is the same." I think this should be true as a style motto for each of us. Everything you touch should bear your imprint. Style is part of what defines "Brand You," and in expressing yourself, every gesture is a statement, so make your mark.

> "Style is part of you, trends are something you wear."
>
> —Donna Karan, designer

What's Your Style Compass?

Great style begins within with an unapologetic appreciation of who you are! This is what impacts how you look, what you wear, and how you wear it. It's also based on your personal desires and how you live your life. Great style is not based on a dress size or an income; it's also not about the trendy. As an editor, I've laughed my way through it bags, it shoes, the latest runway looks, and more, and I'll tell you this: if you really want to define your style, don't get sidetracked. Yves Saint Laurent put it so succinctly when he said, "Trends come and go, but style is eternal," and though there's nothing wrong with giving a nod to the trends, it's so not about being wed to them. Why invest in anything that has a seasonal expiration date written all over it? Real style is based on a bankable wardrobe that is composed of well-defined pieces, plain and simple. This is a strategy everyone can work with as it calls for you to define a style sensibility that's authentically you and works for how you want to express yourself. Once you establish this, it will simplify your life, give order to your closet, and allow you to shop at all price points and dress with confidence.

> " Style is something each of us already has. All we need to do is find it."
> —Diane von Furstenberg, designer

There's nothing more captivating than a gal whose sense of style is so on point that she doesn't think twice about the process. Take, for example, former First Lady Michelle Obama—she never exits the lane of her signature "classic with a twist" style. She's defined a bankable wardrobe composed of sensational dresses and separates that work across the board in her life and come from such diverse retailers as J.Crew and Asos to the top designers in the world. A clear sense of style holds true for eclectic dressers Erykah Badu and Janelle Monáe, who you'll always find in the lane of what appears to be "creative license" but, in reality, is based on a signature theme. For Badu, that means oversize silhouettes, artistic color, pattern mixes, and larger-than-life accessories. Monáe favors retro-esque masculine/feminine separates based on a black-and-white theme and likes building out the look with wide-brimmed hats or her signature Afro-esque crown. Iman oozes glamour, whether dazzling on the red carpet in a designer gown or dashing to lunch in a curvy jacket and jeans. The effortlessly chic Queen Latifah is a classic, and for her stylist, Timothy Snell, the "Man Behind the Curves," as he's known in the industry, that's deliberate. "I'm always looking to have her appear sleek and unfussy, in looks that stand the test of time," says the busy style expert and audience fave known for dispensing curvy-girl know-how on his former Centric TV show *Curvy Style with Timothy Snell*.

" **M**ake sure the things you love serve you well because you have to put them on and serve!"
—Pamela Macklin, wardrobe expert

Yours Truly favors a "classic with a twist" style sensibility and can usually be found in a good frock, even on off days, where a denim dress usually fits the bill. You might see me working a classic sheath dress on camera, but it will always have that unexpected detail that makes the defining difference, e.g., an industrial zipper, a double hem, or a tech fabric. Work often sees me mic'd, whether for TV or at a podium, so Macklin, whom I work with both personally and professionally, makes sure I'm in a dress with a great neckline for what she calls "the strap shot," because the focus on camera is always on the upper body. My style sensibility holds true from head to toe. I might work a pump on any given day, but the shape, the hue, or the texture must have a degree of edge, like my basic pump that's so unbasic in powder blue calf-hair. I love a distinct point of view when it comes to style because it's so easy to reinterpret again and again. I think that's part of the joy of getting dressed. Establishing a clear style ID is a game changer, one that makes all the difference in the world to your confidence and your life, as well as your wallet. To help set your style compass, here are several categories that will help determine what works best for you:

⊚ **Classic:** A true traditionalist who appreciates smart, chic, timeless silhouettes.

- **Classic with a *twist*:** Favors classic pieces with an edge; loves unexpected details, fabrications, hues, and pairing the unexpected.

- **Elegant:** Distinguished by polished, pulled-together, ladylike silhouettes and refined femininity.

- **Glamorous:** Strikes in the bold and the daring, works a high-fashion flair and sensuous designs—think "more is more."

- **Eclectic:** Always the mix master, relishes combining the unpredictable with quirky panache; a true nontraditionalist.

- **Minimalist:** Consistently favors simplicity, clean lines, modern silhouettes, immaculate tailoring, impeccable fabrics, and an overall "less is more" approach.

Closet Confidential

Once you've determined your style sensibility, it's time to define your "bankable wardrobe" by evaluating what works and what doesn't. Macklin is of the mind-set that your closet is an extension of who you are and compares it to relationships. "You have to identify your best friends—in this case, it's the things you turn to all the time. You must also identify your frenemies, the things that are just hanging there for no good reason or those pieces that you don't feel comfortable in," she says. A lot of times we don't like to let go, and that's where she says we get into trouble. "They were good at one time, but they betrayed you, they became tight on your tummy, snug on your hips, and they're not your friends anymore, but you want to keep them around anyway," she says in the midst of a good laugh. On tour, I tell attendees to have a "closet confidential" conversation in front of their clothes and make it known that "some of you will not be moving forward with me!" It's best to be honest and, at the very least, think of editing your closet as an exit strategy that will allow you to be on point. Create three piles: (1) clothing and accessories that will be donated to charity, (2) those that need repairs, and (3) "toss," for those pieces that aren't salvageable. Be brutal with the "toss" pile. If memories are attached, take a picture! Don't equate timeless with old. If something is fraying, has pills or multiple moth holes, say goodbye. Reweaving moth holes is pricey and not worth it unless it's a real investment piece. It costs on average about $25 to $50 to repair each pea-size hole on a cashmere sweater. So don't think twice; you could invest in a new sweater for the cost of your repair. Many of us are guilty of holding onto the past, or waiting for that someday when we return to the size we were five years ago. Don't do this. Now take stock of what remains and determine how these selects will work and decide what needs altering or can be reworked to fit your look.

Good Sport

Give your insecurities to charity! Donate anything that doesn't fit properly (read: it's beyond alteration) to an organization like Dress for Success (www.dressforsuccess.org) because it's time for someone else to enjoy it.

Don't get hung up on your dress size. Like age, it's just a number!

Mikki-ism

POWER POINT

No matter what her style sensibility, behind every well-dressed
woman is a tightly edited closet composed of transformative pieces
that fit like a dream.

It's no mystery. The secret to looking great and dressing with ease
relies on two support systems: a good tailor and a well-ordered closet. A
good tailor should be part of your management team, and you should
have one who can make the kind of magic that extends beyond basic
alterations. The best tailors intuitively recognize your best fit, where
garments should be nipped and tucked or released; they can also alter
necklines and sleeves, determine where your best hemline should fall,
and more. They should also be your go-to when buying "off the rack,"
even the best pieces in store usually leave a little something to be desired. They "almost fit," or need tapering, or a little adjustment here
and there to make them dream-worthy. In between sizes? What I've
learned from experts like Macklin, who provides wardrobe direction to
a number of high-profile women, is that it's best to go up a size when
shopping and then visit a tailor, or have the store's in-house seamstress
customize a fit just for you. Like you, I don't have time to stress how I
look or spend my day fidgeting in something that doesn't fit well, so I
give my concerns to my tailor because empowered women don't make
allowances for designer shortcomings!

I don't know about fashion therapy, but a well-ordered wardrobe of bankable or evergreen pieces certainly makes me feel good. Hey, guilty as charged!

Mikki-ism

I think every gal's closet should be a reflection of her style where everything clicks with everything else, not only affording her the ease of getting dressed quickly but also inspiring her with curated options on what to wear, wherever she's headed. What I know for sure is that it's not about having a closet full of clothes it's about having options you can count on and having them organized in a way that you can choose them effortlessly. There's no time like the present to purchase closet organizers, appropriate hangers, and large trash bags for discards. Personally I hang my clothing by color so I can easily see how I want to pull a look together. You might be a gal who organizes her closet by silhouette in terms of categories, e.g., blouses with blouses, pants with pants. The main idea here is to get and stay organized. Get into the practice of storing your shoes in shoe boxes and placing screenshots or labels on the fronts so you can identify them at a glance. Place handbags in protective cloth bags to protect them from dust, stuffed to retain their shape with enough acid-free tissue paper to stand up on their own, and placed on the shelves along with your jeans and sweaters. Hanging jewelry organizers with clear pockets will keep your best finds like earrings and rings at the ready. I use a glass-top curio for my necklaces and a raw silk covered mannequin to hold/

display my brooches, making my "get ready" a breeze. Today's furniture stores also carry charming jewelry chests with pull-out draws and fitted hooks for all your finds. You can also find great vintage lingerie chests at flea markets that can hold your jewelry on a velvet tray as well, which I think are so befitting of a Queen. Doesn't matter whether your pieces are real or faux, you don't want them to get scratched or lose stones or become tangled and break, so be creative and resourceful in storing them.

Now here's a final word for all closet chicsters:

⊙ Clutter is your enemy. It creates chaos and unnecessary style challenges, so stay organized.

⊙ Choose hangers that allow all your clothing to be displayed at the same level, even if your closet is divided into sections.

⊙ Store off-season pieces in space-saving vacuum packs so your closet isn't overcrowded and you won't have to steam or iron your pieces every time you're ready to get dressed.

⊙ Bonus: Glam up your space! Drop a fierce lighting fixture from the ceiling—new or vintage, place a beautiful rug on the floor or line your closet with an amazing wallpaper. The idea here is to have fun and personalize it by making it engaging and really special.

66 F ashion has always been a repetition of ideas, but what makes it new is the way you put it together."

—Carolina Herrera, designer

Second That

If you're not having fun getting dressed, then what's the point? I'm amused and inspired by Karl Lagerfeld, creative director of such fashion houses as Chanel, Fendi, and his own eponymous label. Lagerfeld excels at newness based on a theme, reinterpreting classics year after year to look modern and fresh. The joy of a bankable wardrobe is the ability to wear what you love again and again. Anchor your look with investment-worthy pieces that can be reinterpreted with a fresh eye and a well-rounded assortment of mileage-making accessories. With your investment pieces in place, you can then add chic, inexpensive finds to the mix to multiply your options on looking fabulous and being frugal! This is how a Queen maximizes her fashion budget, builds a great wardrobe, and always conveys great style.

Fashion Dossier

Create your own "look book" right on your phone or tablet by taking a "selfie" every time you work a look you love. This can also be done on Stylebook, an app that allows you to import your pieces, and add individual picks into magazine-like layouts. Explore new wardrobe combos with what's already in your closet.

When it comes to style, don't put a period where you should put an exclamation mark!

Mikki-ism

Shop Talk

Creating a well-defined wardrobe isn't complicated when you have a strategy in place. When I first started my tenure at *Essence* in the fashion and beauty department, I was on the fashion side and was responsible for selecting fabrics for the pattern houses to create clothing to include on our fashion pages as many sisters made their own style picks. I also handled accessories for our shoots. I always shopped with the specific story in mind, and though the market was full of amazing finds, sticking to the angle of the story is what kept me focused, and therein lies the secret to smart shopping: stick to your story. This will help you know exactly what to buy—that which adds value to your style story—and avoid picks that don't. In order to avoid impulse buys, have a clear idea of your budget and what you need *before* you shop. Listen, shopping isn't referred to as an experience without good reason. The retail environment is set up to entertain you, and when you're browsing without a purpose, it can be challenging. "With the proliferation of e-commerce, retailers are doing more to entice and delight you because they recognize the competition, so when you go into the stores, they're spritzing you with perfume, offering to help you try on a dress, sending for undergarments and/or offering you coffee or tea," Macklin says. This can be quite seductive, so know your purpose for hitting the stores before you go. Make a shopping list at the beginning of each season, jot down what you need first, especially anything that falls in the investment category, and shop accordingly. I hit the stores seasonally and purchase my wardrobe fill-ins and accessory updates in silhouettes that work for me but are instantly thrust "on" by an interesting color, texture, or cut. This allows me to pair with or add on to existing pieces building on a wardrobe that's always current but totally in my lane. If you find that staying focused is challenging, Macklin suggests shopping online or at least saving your receipts for recovery! I often peruse sites that sell a lifestyle or an experience versus just clothing like Net-a-Porter and MatchesFashion. I also review online the New York, Paris, London, and Milan collections of those designers who tell a story for style ideas—and then go shopping in my closet with a newly inspired mind-set!

Style is a story, and it really comes down to how you want to express yourself. Working with some of the best stylists in the business on shoots, I find inspiration everywhere, from old movies to exotic destinations; from the compelling street style of the most divine sisters in Harlem in their patternalia mixes to the *Dolce Vita*–inspired style of women in Portofino, Italy, where a circle skirt paired with a T-shirt, ballet flats, and killer eardrops transports me to the chic-dom of the '50s. Designer Stella Jean, whose Creole heritage and brilliant work with Haitian and African artisans continuously inspires. Her collections can be found on such sites as Farfetch and MatchesFashion. Also inspirational to the point of pearl clutching is Nigerian-born designer Duro Olowu, whose innovative designs mix patterns, textiles, and vibrant prints that translate into wearable art. His distinctive pieces can be found on some of the best-dressed women I know, from Michelle Obama to Solange Knowles, and at such destination sites as Lyst, MatchesFashion, and Farfetch.

I've been inspired in many a legendary bookstore, trapped in bygone eras as I visualized style ideas for a shoot (or, selfishly, for my closet!). I'm not alone in this passion. Tim (Timothy Snell), as I affectionately call him, loves Galignani's bookstore in Paris, France, a beloved resource for the cognoscenti. There we were one afternoon shopping to our hearts' content when in walks designer Karl Lagerfeld. We were amused as "Kaiser Karl" moved through the aisles with his entourage of assistants, tapping his books of choice with a grand fan! Stylists and designers alike take their inspiration from books, travel, the theater, cultures, history, icons, and more. Celebrity stylist Susan Moses, author of *The Art of Dressing Curves: The Best Kept Secrets of a Fashion Stylist*, takes inspiration from art, music, and such sites as *Fashion Bomb Daily* and *Glamour*, but she's also inspired by those she calls "curvy connoisseurs," top bloggers whose sites are full of style tips and the latest news. Moses, whose clients include Jill Scott, Brandy, Kathy Bates, and Wynonna Judd, believes in the power of self-awareness and self-acceptance above all. "When you know your body type and you are armed with confidence, you can open the pages of mainstream fashion magazines, be inspired by the latest runway looks or fashion sites and more, as I have been doing for years," concludes the tall, curvaceous beauty!

Always choose quality over quantity, but do buy quality in multiples!

Mikki-ism

Always filter your buys through your style sieve. "You should be looking to buy items that work back to the clothing in your existing wardrobe. It's never about buying something for a moment or a stand-alone piece," Macklin adds. Invest your money on what you wear the most. For example: black pants, pumps, a coat, or whatever's big on rotation or repeated wear in your life should be of the best quality your money can buy. When you find a great silhouette, do buy it in multiples as this will save you time as well as extend the life of your wardrobe. The same holds true for those "fillers" (white shirts, black turtlenecks, etc.) and moderate to frugal finds that may or may not be seasonal. Empowered with knowing your style story, you'll be able to shop high and low price points with ease. This is a savvy move that women both in and out of the spotlight work to their advantage. When it comes to nailing great finds, it's more about your eye and sense of style than your budget. You don't need the so-called confidence of high price tags or designer labels to convince yourself that your look works. I've seen many a gal who forked over a bundle for big-ticket labels but still lacked great style. The sharper your sense of personal style, the more you'll know exactly when to invest and when to save, and avoid being duped. There's nothing like the thrill of buying an investment pick and then throwing in a steal that gives a nod to the trends. With mainstream retailers and trends-at-a-price destinations like Zara, now snagging the seasons look doesn't have to break the bank. However, no matter the price tag, always stick with what works for your style sensibility. Don't ever make the mistake of changing your style in an effort to pull out all the stops. Be you! Here's the last word on how to maximize your shopping experience:

- Know when to shop: Fashion is an ever-evolving business, and some designers are offering immediate buys post their ready-to-wear shows. But instant gratification aside, you'll need a shopping strategy for the best results. (1) If you're an online shopper, sign up for email notices to your favorite sites. This helps ensure that when "new arrivals" come in you get first picks before your size is sold out. If you like hitting the stores, identify a salesperson who can help you with your best buys as well as alert you to upcoming sales. For new destinations, be there when the doors open, when there's less traffic; chances are you'll have a salesperson all to yourself. (2) Be aware of merchandise deliveries so you don't miss out. In general, spring fashion begins arriving in store in February and is in full throttle by March. Come June, as you're beginning to think about outdoor parties, early fall picks begin appearing. By August, fall is in, and close on its heels are the most glittering holiday finds. Plan accordingly. For example, if you're in need of a great black "forever" clutch, know that between October and November the stores are on overload with items in the accessory and evening departments. So that's the time to buy. Ditto for that LBD you might want to add to your wardrobe. (3) Know about sales *ahead* of time so you can take full advantage of them. Here again, get on the email lists for retailers you frequent or want to watch so you'll get notifications of pending sales, coupons, and/or special discounts for both in-store and online use.

⦿ Cultivate relationships with salespersons who will place your info on file for calls regarding sales and what's new in store.

⦿ Get VIP service: Look to a personal shopper or, again, establish a relationship with a sales associate. When working with a personal shopper, Macklin advises scheduling a consultation first because anyone who's looking to help you has to be interested in your story in order to add value. "Make sure the person conveys an understanding of what you want," she says, adding, "A great personal shopper should look to build a relationship with you before they sell you anything." I schedule time with the sales associates at the places I frequent, as a result, the ladies always have my fitting room ready with selects personalized for me. I also email finds to Macklin for input prior to any purchases. This practice saves time and money.

⦿ Keep your credit card on file: I'm a big believer in the practice of "charge and send," as it helps me avoid waiting in line, something I just haven't mastered yet. It's a good practice for those stores you trust and where you have a great salesperson or personal shopper at the ready.

66 **M**y mission in life is not merely to survive, but to thrive; and to do so with some passion, some compassion, some humor, and some style."

—Dr. Maya Angelou, poet, author, civil rights activist

Defining a Bankable Wardrobe: The Essentials

No matter your style persona, every gal can build a wardrobe that embodies her own look and feel. With the right pieces you'll never have to worry about what to wear again. You'll also avoid "occasion shopping," which is always stressful and costly. Given that you're managing life, family, work, your social life, and more, having basic core pieces in your closet make getting dressed a joy and can be best counted on for replays because they can be reinterpreted from season to season. Remember, your goal is to dress in a way that conveys great personal style, so make your list and check it twice!

Frock Stars

It Figures

The allure of a great dress is never to be underestimated, and the options are endless. Best buys are those in the most womanly fabrics that "stretch," "move," or "shape," and the difference allows you to take getting dressed from "okay" to "wow" in minutes! Think of a great dress as a key part of your bankable wardrobe, and aim for great necklines (from the classic V- or jewel neck to a great boatneck, a faux wrap, or a scoop neck), several clean cuts, and/or variations on a silhouette that clicks every time, and you've got one of the MVPs of great style. For sure you'll want to anchor your wardrobe with dresses that are flexible in that they allow you to change up their persona with a switch of accessories.

Takeaway

Two to three great dresses in seasonless fabrics and solid, nonseasonal hues that keep pace with your lifestyle and have the ability to move from day to night.

Go on and add zest to your LBD with a conversation-worthy shoe, a knockout red lipstick, and a ring that turns heads. After all, playing it safe is so overrated!

Mikki-ism

The LBD

There's no greater style star than the little black dress, as it's a smart investment pick and a wardrobe powerhouse with plenty of attitude. No matter the season, it's the most seamless way to transition from day to night as it never fails to deliver maximum impact with minimal effort. Again, think great necklines, quality fabrics that stand repeated wear, and cuts that flatter you coming and going, be it a minimalist sheath with an impeccable fit that goes from the boardroom to a business dinner, a simple cut fit-and-flare that appears with a cardi by day and heads off to a great reception solo by night, or a fly wrap dress that goes from work to an art gallery. There's nothing more perennially chic than the LBD, and the smartest buys will become great girlfriends who are always on standby for any occasion. Here's how to make the most of this investment:

- Be willing to spend a little more for this forever-reliable piece so it stands the test of time.

- Avoid LBDs with jeweled or embellished necklines as there's no room for reinterpretation.

◉ Choose a reputable dry cleaner so the fabric doesn't take a beating and come back shiny and stressed out!

◉ Maintain your LBD like any piece that you wear repeatedly by checking the hem and examining it for deodorant stains or spots so it's impeccable and always ready to go.

Takeaway

A little black dress is like a good girlfriend who never lets you down. Make it a point to have at least one good dress that you can count on no matter what the invitation reads, that's so versatile it can be dressed up with heels or dressed down with flats.

66 **P**eople will stare. Make it worth their while."
—Harry Winston, jeweler

This Bud's for You

I love a "happy dress," and I've found there's nothing like a hothouse floral dress to bring a smile to your face and add a statement to your wardrobe! Impactful flower prints, whether on a black, white, or zesty-hued background, give new life and loads of whimsy to timeless silhouettes without being trendy. When you're shopping, keep your eye out for those with the kind of distinction that you'll love forever. And you know what? If they say, "Notice me," so what? It's not a uniform!

Takeaway

Get your print works on, as there's a floral wonder for everyone in the bunch.

Maximize the Moment

A beautiful maxi dress always looks pulled together. Whether paired with a great boot or a flat sandal, it's no-brainer dressing that works for any style persona. In the right fabric, it's a year-round pick that's ready to go whether you're hitting festivals, going out to dinner, or having the girls over on a wintry night. When entertaining at home, I find it doesn't get any easier or more comfortable, for that matter, and I keep my eye out for the best in flow at destinations that range from Net-a-Porter and Zara to Nordstrom and Neiman Marcus, to name a few. Maxi dresses also travel quite well and offer Yours Truly some of the best options for island dwelling. Come winter, I look for those in soft matte jersey as they're perfect for curling up with a good book on snowy evenings or when friends come to dinner. Depending on the silhouette, they're also the perfect pick when you've had a good meal and need a little "hide-and-chic." And you thought making an effort was complicated!

Takeaway

To splurge or not to splurge. This is a pick that can be as easy on the budget as you want it to be, so if you're not already engaged, try one on and imagine the possibilities!

Cardi Show

Nothing beats a jewel-neck cardigan as a polished player in one's closet as it's the best pick your money can buy. I'm always on the lookout for this style staple to take me through the year in various weights (cotton, cashmere, merino), hues, even various textures. Of course, my black cardis get worked the most, so I tend to buy these in multiples. Cardis work over everything, are a great layering piece, go day to night, can be dressed up or down, and even worn backwards, which I do by pairing one over a chic pencil skirt. I also like to hit the vintage shops for distinctive buttons as this is another fun way to change the persona and take it from basic to sensational. While other types of cardis have their place, none possess such chic simplicity as the jewel neck, and in today's retail landscape, you can purchase a great cardi in all weights, shades, sizes, and prices. Worth noting: make sure it fits well, and steer clear of those that are cut too full to avoid looking like a dated librarian! Cozy, but not good.

Takeaway

One black or camel cardigan equals versatility, timeless appeal, a great layering piece, and your year-round player for work, casual weekends, and more.

Pant Logic

A well-cut pair of pants or slacks in quality, wrinkle resistant fabric (stretch wools, tropical woolens, or microfiber) is a moneyed wardrobe staple that works across the board. In general, I find flared flat-front pants with a floor-skimming hem or boot-cut pants are sleek, nearly universal styles for most body shapes and the most versatile as they work with a multiplicity of jackets and tops. They also move well from workday to dressy nights. Slim, flat-front pants (minus the vertical side pockets that stick out) that hit slightly above or below the ankle are quite chic and multitask well. And when they have a degree of stretch, or control, like those by Alfani, which are available in regular and plus sizes, they shape and flatter. Also consider adding a tuxedo pant with minimal detailing (no belt tabs) as a smart take on evening dressing. Trousers, on the other hand, can be daunting, depending on your height, body shape, and size, so I recommend having them sized to fit well by a tailor. When shopping, you'll want to make sure they are sufficiently roomy in the crotch and, if you're a curvy girl, that they don't add too much volume by way of pleats and pockets. Great pant resources for curvy girls include such retailers as Macy's, Nordstrom, Lane Bryant, and Lafayette 148.

Takeaway
Basic priority: two pairs of black pants that are such a snap you can pair them with everything. And note, when you find a style that works, don't hesitate to invest in multiple pairs.

Play the Blues
Denim has undergone a complete overhaul with the entry of designers who have changed the playing field and brought innovative styling, improved quality, and more options for women with real bodies to jeans and denim separates. Denim has also been reimagined for use in footwear and accessories, living up to its all-around player status. With companies like CJ by Cookie Johnson, NYDJ, and James Jeans, as well as curve-specific retailers offering reality-checked brands, women of color can now find the perfect pair of jeans that offers style, shape, comfort, and cool, and that is also polished enough to go into the workplace. As with pants, you'll want to identify the right cut when choosing jeans so you always look pulled together. Don't get caught up on sizes; pay attention to cut, fit, quality, and color. Options abound, from straight leg, skinny, boot cut, and flares to boyfriend and capris, but again, it's best to determine which cut(s) fit you well, work in your life, and can be paired with items in your existing wardrobe to create versatility. Shaping is everything, and whether it's through the tummy support of a high or wide waistband or the seaming that lifts your rear or sculpts your thighs, the jeans you wear should be so fabulous that you don't think twice about slipping them on. Shape aside, I prefer those that have a degree of stretch as I think style and comfort go hand in hand. I also like a dark denim or black as they fit my "classic with a twist" sensibility and

transition well from day to night. Great denim jackets and skirts also represent options that you can work into your wardrobe to add flair, texture, and freshness. A smart denim pump represents yet another way to play the jean game and adds some whimsy to your coterie of great looks. Think of your denim pump as a noncompete player and pair it with dresses, pants, skirts, etc. Just don't match it with other denim separates as it's about mixing, not matching. Besides, you're far more creative than that!

Takeaway

Though an all-around staple, mixing denim in a modern wardrobe goes way beyond a great pair of jeans, so aside from choosing the mainstay cut that you love, consider experimenting with denim outside of its designated role.

Skirting the Issue

The flair of a sharp skirt is a good core piece around which to style. When it comes to this wardrobe staple, I think every gal should own the perfect black pencil in a seasonless fabric, which can be purchased at all price points and be styled to suit all of your best-dressed needs. Fit is key. Translation: it should fit across your hips without pulling. Here enlist a tailor to make sure it fits properly at the waist and to taper or peg it at the bottom so it's not too boxy. Best buys are those in a suiting fabric like a lightweight gabardine that's lined or one of the many fabrications with a hint of stretch. Once this basic is in place, consider adding a black lace pencil skirt as an alternative evening option. Pleats, flares, flounced, gored, trumpet, or A-line skirts also present options that can round out your wardrobe but will depend on your style sensibility as well as your figure. All in all, fabrics rule, and hemlines count immensely as they do have the ability to impact your style statement. For example, let's say you've purchased a black pencil skirt at a steal of a price, only to find that when you wear it, every crease or wrinkle stays put throughout the day, making you look far less polished than when you left the house. Not good! Or you might be the gal who bought a full midcalf skirt thinking that it would look great with a pair of heels, but instead it makes you look frumpy. Best solutions: look at fabric content and pay attention to silhouettes and hemlines; always take a basic heel and a flat with you when shopping in store to get a sense of what has real-life potential and what doesn't.

Takeaway

Nail your versatile basic black pencil skirt in a quality fabric and an impeccable fit first, then make any additions based on how well they'll round out your wardrobe.

Top Priority

Dressing well is about choosing the smartest separates to boost your wardrobe mileage and make your every style move a fab, effortless experience. Tops are the workhorses of your wardrobe, as they allow you to pull together a look with ease as well as lend newness to existing pieces. You can play with color, texture, prints, and a range of fabrics. Here's the checklist:

- **Shirts:** A white button-down. Depending on your style sensibility, this could be a forever classic, a French cuff, or a crisp '50s-inspired shirt with three-quarter sleeves. Do make sure that it's fitted as much as your comfort factor will allow.

- **Blouses:** Whether soft and feminine, chic and sophisticated, or bold and edgy, a few good blouses that "play well with others" in your wardrobe of separates is a must. They represent an easy way to add color, prints, and personality while moving your look through the workweek and beyond with ease.

- **Turtlenecks/sweaters:** It doesn't get any more smart and sophisticated than the classic black turtleneck. Here again, depending on your style sensibility, you can move from classic to edgy just by the shape of a sleeve or the fabric and texture. It's worth stocking up on them in different weights—from cashmere to cotton to neoprene—in a sublime fit. Camel or navy also represent good mixer options. Sweater dressing overall is a modern way to build a wardrobe of substance. Think pieces that complete or transform a look, like a luxe sweater coat that works over dresses and separates or a classic V-neck that not only chases the chill but pairs well with a jean on the weekend and slips over a pant for work come Monday.

- **Tees:** Be they playful, business casual, or simply essential layering pieces, a few terrific tees are all you need to complete a look in seconds.

Takeaway

Tops form the essential basics of any prized wardrobe, and that means having the kind of choices that allow you to mix and match to your heart's content. Bottom line: stock up on the pieces you wear most frequently and, where possible, make sure they are washable to cut down on dry cleaning costs.

It's a Cinch

Jackets represent the great collaborators in a bankable wardrobe. A well-cut blazer will extend your wardrobe and add versatility to your repertoire of looks. It's best to opt for polished hues such as black or navy that speak to your style sensibility. A bonus addition to any wardrobe is a soft glove-leather jacket to work over dresses and separates effortlessly, lending a fresh new attitude every time. When shopping, avoid the trendy picks as you want this item to have real staying power. Instead, look for *twists* on the classic in cut and fabrication, to accentuate your personal style. Have your style basics in place? Then consider those that give a *nod*—key word, "nod"—to the trends, whether in color or shape.

Takeaway
Mileage-making style, practicality, and long-term investment are all to be had by investing in the right jacket. Plan accordingly.

Entrenched
A trench coat is one of the most versatile pieces a gal can own as it instantly pulls a look together come rain or come shine. My first fashion investment was a classic double-breasted Burberry trench with a twist that allowed for it to be buttoned traditionally or buttoned back to remain open. Though the classic trench has undergone many interpretations, its multiseasonal fabric and hue make it nonpareil for all occasions. Trench style translates so well that you can get a great buy at any price point; it just depends on whether you want to make an investment buy or a style buy. It also depends on such factors as where you live, how you like to work it, and how often you'll pop it on. What you'll need to determine is whether you'll want a single or double-breasted version. Color is another consideration and there are many variations. Finally, when purchasing your trench, make sure it fits well over your clothing, consider the length, that the sleeves aren't tight, and, if it's vented in the back, that the vents lie flat. Think of it this way: when all checkpoints are in place, you can forget about how you look, and that's an essential element of a great buy.

Takeaway
A trench coat is a wardrobe MVP and the cornerstone of a well-edited look that takes you everywhere. Choose wisely.

"Sale"? Why, that's my favorite term in any language!

Mikki-ism

Top It Off

A coat is a serious investment, one that should make a statement yet blend seamlessly into your wardrobe. You'll want to analyze your best options carefully based on fabric, shape, and versatility. A good-quality full-length cloth coat is to your wardrobe what an exclamation mark is to a sentence. It should emphasize your point of view, so invest well. It can cost you, but I recommend you do the "cost-per-wear" analogy in terms of how many times you'll work it, and once you see how that adds up, it'll make you smile. Of course, depending on the climate you live in, you'll want to make sure it not only serves your style requirements but keeps you warm in the process. And don't settle. A lot of times it's best to wait for a sale so you can get the coat you really want and stay within your budget. While I love a classic slim style with a twist, I also favor A-line silhouettes due to their ladylike flair. A wrap is an all-time classic. Another great wardrobe option is a three-quarter-length coat as it works well over pencil skirts, pants, and jeans and in the right hue can also work for evening. The point is, you don't have to settle for a basic buy; instead buy the coat that suits your basic needs and build your options by adding to it.

Takeaway

This is a real fashion investment, one that should be special yet versatile enough to work over everything in your wardrobe.

66 "B e authentic! Master those silhouettes that are
amazing on you!"

—Timothy Snell, celebrity stylist

Having a Ball

Dressing to celebrate your figure should be one of your most thrilling in-
dulgences! Got great arms? Work them in sleeveless frocks and divine tops.
Possess great legs? Go for those hemlines that shape or move, coupled
with conversation-worthy shoes. Whittled waistline? Make it count with
eye-catching belts, fitted jackets, and curve-conscious dresses. Need I say
more?

Strong Suit: Swimwear Magic

Whether you favor a great one-piece, a '50s-inspired high-waisted
two-piece, the perfect bikini, or a minimalist tankini, you'll want to
spring for a look that's flattering, comfortable, and striking—water
optional! "When buying a swimsuit, open your eyes up to the possibilities—think vibrant color, great lines, and fun picks," says the
designer of the Timothy Snell Swimwear Collection with Always for
Me. Fit is key, so don't get hung-up on the numbers; try on different
sizes to find your best fit. The biggest mistake you can make is to buy
a swimsuit that's too small or too big. Think about how you'll put
your swimsuit to use: Are you a poolside gal who's simply looking
for fun in the sun or one who surfs like there's no tomorrow? How
often will you take it out for a swim? Once you've determined your

goal, shop with your body type in mind so you can take the plunge
with ease.

For example, if you're small-busted, think padding, demi cups
that lift and create cleavage, or detailing elements like ruffles or
embellishments. If you need help "bringing up the rear," so to
speak, it's all about shaping and ruching. If you're on the thin
side, look to suits that give the illusion of curves with shaping
and padding. If fit is still an issue, experts recommending shopping at swimwear boutiques or lingerie stores that carry swimsuits, as this is where a bra specialist can help you find your most
flattering picks.

In Tim's book, curvy girls should look for the following: under-
wires for support, zippers for control, silhouettes that don't cut
your thighs; wide straps or halters and ruching and tucking,
which are essential to shaping and defining areas, especially the
waistline. Before you book that vacation or staycation, here are
some brands and resources to consider:

- Always for Me
- Athleta
- J.Crew
- Miraclesuit
- Inches Off
- Eloquii
- Torrid
- Gottex
- Monif C.
- Michael Kors
- Norma Kamali
- Eres

- La Blanca
- Everything But Water
- Dillard's
- Lane Bryant

Winning Undercover

Every Queen needs an array of great underpinnings that, like makeup, look like you, only better. I've found that if it weren't for the right lingerie, half of my clothes could never leave the closet! Now, I'm all for the sexy picks—give me the red lace bra or a nude silk chemise—but I'm also about the pieces that shrink, shape, smooth, and "don't tell" that they're on duty or why! Here, then, are those "undercover agents" and support strategies that enhance your presentation:

- Make it a point to go for a yearly bra fitting as measurements do change and it's essential to have the right support. Oftentimes we shop according to cup size without taking into account the importance of the right fit around our rib cage and the back. An expert will take this into consideration along with how securely the straps fit as well as whether the bridge of the bra sits flush against your breastbone. You can also try companies like True&Co. (True&Co.com), where you can assess your perfect fit via an online quiz that determines your cup size, breast shape, and fit and be directed to your best options. You can buy direct from the site as well as use their Home Try-On program, which will ship bras to you for just that.

- Bag those bras that move through your wardrobe and meet your needs. Your checklist could include a molded sweater bra, a seamless essential to wear under T-shirts and sweaters; a strapless/convertible bra to wear with halters, strapless dresses, and garments that have thin straps; a demi or low-cut bra for plunging necklines; sport bras for support in and out of the gym; and a push-up or balconette bra for times when you want that extra lift. Then indulge your "sexy" and go for the lacy, frilly, flirty, and whatever else makes you feel extra special—just make sure it has the best support your money can buy. Finally, keep in mind that bras, like anything else, have an expiration date, so do plan to replace them within the year.

◉ Assess your shaping desires. Select the body shapers that give you a smooth and slimming fit, from spandex bikers and bodysuits to waist shapers, tanks, and slips.

◉ Pick hues accordingly. Invest in the basics of nude and black first. (I'm always on the lookout for chocolate or woody browns that blend seamlessly with my complexion under light clothing.) Then spring for the colors you love as we all want to have a little fun. Fill in. Get your all-around bottom basics—seamless briefs, boy shorts, high-rise and low-rise thongs (if that's you)—and silicone or adhesive bras (molded to adhere to your body) for backless styles; cutlets/inserts (to fill and push up), great for plunging necklines; silicone cups, also perfect for backless styles; double-stick tape strips (to keep clothing in place where needed, e.g., plunging necklines), etc.

Cover your bases: if you've got that garment for which you need the perfect underpinnings and you're unsure of what fills the bill, take it into the store and a good sales associate in the lingerie department will be all be too happy to suggest options that work.

66 **W**hen it comes to lingerie, have your measurements in hand, be clear about your body type, what your shape-enhancing and support concerns are, and please don't be intimidated by seaming."

—Susan Moses, celebrity stylist

Taking Shape

Whether shopping bra basics or frill-seeking pieces that break the mold, here's your resource checklist:

Global Retailers
- La Perla
- Agent Provocateur
- Victoria's Secret

Nationwide Retailers
- Nordstrom
- Bloomingdale's
- Macy's

Online Destinations
- HerRoom.com
- Anita.com
- Wacoal-America.com
- CurvyKate.com
- BareNecessities.com
- Bravissimo.com
- AdoreMe.com
- Asos.com
- HipsAndCurves.com

- ClassicShapewear.com
- CurvyCouture.com
- AffinitasIntimates.com
- ThirdLove.com

Laid Bare

Talk about a feminine flourish. If you're lingerie obsessed or a bride to be, think pretty, sexy, cool, and don't miss these Big Apple destinations or at least their sites:

Journelle
125 Mercer Street
New York, NY 10012
212-255-7803
Journelle.com

La Petite Coquette
51 University Place
New York, NY 10003
212-473-2478
TheLittleFlirt.com

Sugar Cookies
122 W. 20th Street
New York, NY 10011
212-242-6963
SugarCookiesNYC.com

Agent Provocateur
133 Mercer Street
New York, NY 10012
212-965-0229
AgentProvocateur.com

Town Shop
2270 Broadway
New York, NY 10024
212-724-8160
TownShop.com

It's All in the Mix

RSVP in Style!

Conquer the night and your "what to wear" fears by adhering to the pieces that flatter you and allow you to have a great time without having second thoughts about how you look. Think of any invitation as a time to look special while giving a nod to the occasion. Ask yourself: Who's hosting the event? What is the nature of the occasion? Where will it take place? Answering questions like these always help me define my choices. My wardrobe revolves primarily around dresses, so I don't reinvent the wheel when it's time to step out. If it's an after-work event, I reach for a dress that effortlessly transitions from day to night. If the occasion calls for "festive attire," I pick a party dress that moves. Perhaps you're a separates fashionista. If so, play sensuous picks that work overtime, such as a sensational pantsuit with a glam tee that will go the distance, or a romantic blouse that charms a pencil skirt, or a fluid pant that easily steps well into the night with a sexy sandal. Afternoon wedding? Think festive frocks or a sophisticated pantsuit or jumpsuit, but nothing that will upstage the bride. If it's a black-tie event, know that there are always other options to a traditional gown—many a georgette maxi dress can hit the scene with the right accessories and do what it's supposed to. You could make your entrance in a fab tuxedo, so don't stress it. Do you, and have a great time!

Hosiery Logic

Long before control-top panty hose, my mother wore silk stockings with fancy garter belts. I loved watching her sit on the edge of the bed or her sitting room ottoman as she slipped into her stockings and hooked them in place. This could be why I'm so panty hose adverse. Personally, I prefer thigh-highs as I love the diverse array of styles and the modern technology that allows them to adhere to your body, which means no more garter belts. In the spring, I favor fine fishnets in skintone hues till temps warm up enough for bare legs and microfiber black opaques in winter. But, thigh-high's aren't for everyone and today's pantyhose offer high-functioning shaping capabilities and an array of style, color, and texture options. Here are my go-to labels and resources:

- Spanx
- Hue
- Wolford
- Fogal
- Hanes
- Gaetano Cazzola
- Hosieree.com

Bank on It: Highly Fashionable Things Every Gal Should Own

Accessories are a passion worth indulging as they express your point of view and instantly transform a look into anything you want it to be in nano-seconds. They also add great mileage to your wardrobe and carry a look from season to season, day to night, fun to sophisticated, and more. What should be on your "most-wanted" list are the smartest pieces to amp up your wardrobe and lend a dash of creativity that makes every look uniquely you.

Here's what should be on your list of "insta-glam" picks:

- Diamond or cubic zirconia studs.
- A smart timepiece: An investment piece, be it a traditional timekeeper that adds character or a savvy, up-to-the-moment mobile device with a touchscreen display to help you keep it moving.
- Hoops.
- Cuffs: The best wrist candy to accentuate any look.
- Cocktail rings: Glam-slam additions that work overtime.
- Brooches: Utterly chic, especially when worn in multiples on a coat, a dress, or a jacket.
- Belts: Pulls a look together and makes it stand out in a cinch.

- Scarves: Conversation-worthy prints that can be worn at the neck, nonchalantly tied on a satchel, or on your head and paired with great hoops.
- A transitional clutch: A classic envelope in leather or patent that works day into evening.
- A medium satchel: A first-class bag that's polished, sharp, roomy, and represents you well.
- A multitasking tote: To carry all your needs in great style.
- A versatile pump: Well designed, with low cleavage that clicks with everything; keep it fresh and unexpected, but never go to such heights that you sacrifice comfort for style.
- Nude heels: Your "beauty shoe"! A wear-with-all shoe or sandal in a sister-friendly hue that not only extends your legs but also goes with everything in your closet.
- A classy flat or skimmer: An easy, wear-with-everything pick.
- Metallic sandals: A dazzling touch that instantly glams up every look.
- Black peau de soie pump: A chic pick to move right into the night.

In a Clutch

I think it's hilarious how my day bags are always overweight and my tiny clutches, well, they're on a diet! I'm the girl by day who can't live without this and that (you didn't really think I was going to say "the kitchen sink," did you?), and by night I'm comfortable on "beauty rations." Go figure. I will say this: I've learned from the best in the business concerning what to stash in a clutch. To quote R&B songster Montell Jordan, "This is how we do it!"

- Listerine pack for kissing breath
- Retractable lip brush predaubed with lipstick or gloss
- Mini compact mirror

- BeautyBlender Blotterazzi sponge for zapping shine and checking perspiration without disturbing makeup
- Cell phone—hey, a girl's got to stay in touch, right?

Pin One On

Every girl needs a fab brooch or two that inspires her to have fun and adds that certain je ne sais quoi to her wardrobe. At a pop-up shop, wardrobe expert Pamela Macklin gave new life to old brooches and a few newbies by pinning them on my cloth and fur clutch bags. Now I'm working multiples on coats and dresses or single eye-catchers on the knit skullcaps she customizes, known as "Glammies." Inspired, one night I popped a huge "crystal" spider on the back of a fab black cocktail dress. And you thought playtime was for little girls.

Finishing Touch

I think gloves are the pièce de résistance of a look. Back in the day, my mother and my aunties wouldn't emerge from the house without their white, black, or navy gloves, whether in leather or cotton. When I started covering the ready-to-wear collections in Paris, I would hit glove bars to be fitted for *une paire de gants* (a pair of gloves). Out the gloves would come, thin and flat as a knife, and a conical instrument would be used to open up the fingers before putting them on your hands and making sure they fit to perfection. When shopping for the perfect pair, I want you to think in terms of material, length, color, fit, and use. For certain you'll want your basic black leather pair, and whether they are lined or unlined depends on the climate you live in. The length you choose—wrist, elbow, or opera—should be based on your lifestyle. Beyond black, have fun with color and fabrications, and always look to add the unexpected. I like mesh, cotton, light woolens, and special embellishments and design treatments, and I'm smitten with fingerless shorties for special occasions. I shop everywhere from department stores and vintage havens like The Way We Wore in Los Angeles to one of my favorite retail glove destinations, Sermoneta (www.sermonetagloves.com), as a well-chosen pair of gloves are just too chic to sigh for!

> I'm all about saving for a rainy day—as in money, that is—but not when it comes to a great look. In my book every day is an occasion to style.
>
> *Mikki-ism*

Pop-tastic!

There's nothing like a pop or heady dose of color to make a statement, from jewel tones to brights and pastels. Why not kick the charm of a ladylike LBD into "next" territory by pairing it with an eye-catching pump in sizzling orange suede or a vivid fringed sandal. Push your look forward with a fab satchel in an electric blue. Or team a fab pair of "drops"—read earrings—in zesty orange enamel against a crisp white shirt! Liberate a basic black frock with a yellow cuff. How fresh! Don't hit the snooze button and miss your wardrobe wake-up call.

Hit Refresh

Between work, home duties, and social calls, my schedule is packed enough to require a clone. Quick switches from the office to high-powered dinners and glittering receptions can be a challenge, but I've learned how to make it happen by investing in the following:

- LBDs that move from day to night
- A cocktail dress in a mood-thrilling hue

- Jersey or georgette maxi dresses in a timeless color (black, navy, red, coral) that can double as a gown
- Great separates that can read evening
- Transformative accessories that add mileage to all of the above

Style Equations

When stepping out calls for a little shimmer and shine, do mix the best accessories, but please avoid piling on everything you've got. Also, don't work the necklace with the matching bracelets, earrings, ring, etc.—unless you're getting a check from the manufacturer for advertising! Know when enough is enough and when in doubt, leave something behind for the next occasion. Enough said.

Getaway Chic

Going on holiday? First things first: check Weather.com to see what the temps are at your intended destination then decide what you're doing, where you're going, and who you're seeing. When it's time to pack, create your packing list so you're not toting a million and one pieces and so many bags that your trip costs a fortune in luggage fees. Think smart by choosing items that work well together and allow you to create a wardrobe of great looks with a minimal number of pieces. This is where transformative accessories become the workhorses. Prep by laying your looks out on the bed and snapping them as a reference, this way you can see if there's anything you can leave behind. I often remind myself "you're not running away from home, just going on vacation, because I like to pack a lot options!" Hitting a cold climate? My suggestions include cozy cashmere and jersey separates, great dresses, chic boots, a fur cowl, a down vest, and a few multitasking accessories. Heading to a sun-soaked destination? I like a straw brim to protect my hair color, maxi dresses, swimsuits, and cover-ups that work overtime. According to celebrity stylist Timothy Snell, a great cover-up is everything. "The swimwear cover-ups of today can be worn from the beach to the streets—they are the new key accessories!" he declares. For the international style authority, swimwear cover-ups now reflect the runways of the world, taking on bold color, prints, color blocking, and embellishments so they are *the* contemporary buy. Long before cover-ups moved from functional to fabulous, the gals I know put their summer frocks into play. I'll never forget celebrity makeup artist Fran Cooper (who I worked with on several cover shoots with Janet Jackson) and dolls whose names I cannot share wading into the pool at our wedding in the Catskills. How glamorous they were with their diaphanous dresses floating around them!

Now, before you pack your passport, throw in a travel-size mending kit as well as nail polish remover packets in case you have to smooth a chip. Do make sure you include sanitary supplies just in case you have an early *lady moment* as well. Include a cortisone cream that addresses everything from insect bites to pop-up heat rashes that can occur in steamy climates and an antibiotic ointment if needed for an unexpected scratch or scrape. Finally, don't leave home without a statement-making pair of fierce shades so you can work clean glamour (sparely there makeup) from dawn to dusk. Make sure they cover your eyes completely, including your brows, and frame your look well. My current fave, actress Eva Marcille's utterly fabulous First Ave Eyewear collection—they're right up there with my MAC makeup buys. Travel well.

Insider Style Guide

Calling all "brandistas"! If looking for the must-have fashion brands at a price, chances are they can be found online at one of three types of sites:

1 **Off-price sites:** Offer high-quality designer clothing, accessories, and more at reduced prices.
2 **Flash-sale sites:** Offer specific sales and deals through limited-time events on designer clothes, accessories, home goods, and more; all require membership, though most memberships are free.

3   **Search sites:** Fashion search engines that allow you to find brands, compare pricing and identify the stores where they can be found; if you're looking for a particular item, you can enter the style number or name of the designer and chances are you can find it well below retail pricing.

Off-Price Sites

- **TheOutnet.com:** Clothing, bags, shoes, accessories; over 350 designers with prices up to 75 percent off.
- **6pm.com:** Designer shoes, bags, and clothing (including plus-size options) with new sales and deals daily.
- **Bluefly.com:** High-end designer fashions and accessories for less.

Flash-Sale Sites

- **Gilt.com:** Insider access to top designer labels at up to 70 percent off retail.
- **Zulily.com:** Daily deals up to 70 percent off on women's apparel and accessories.
- **BeyondTheRack.com:** Designer brand apparel and accessories at up to 80 percent off retail.
- **Ruelala.com:** Desired brands at members-only prices, new deals daily.
- **Groupon.com:** Top labels, deep discounts on clothing, shoes, accessories, and more.
- **HauteLook.com:** Daily curated events featuring fashion, accessories, and beauty brands at prices up to 75 percent off.

Search Sites

- **ShopStyle.com:** A fashionable search engine for clothing, shoes, accessories, and beauty.
- **DesignerApparel.com:** Destination engine dedicated to designer apparel and accessories.
- **Lyst.com:** Destination engine for designer and moderate brands featuring clothing (including plus-size options), shoes, and accessories.

Notes to Self...

Notes to Self...

Notes to Self...

7

Master You Inc.

People often debate the possibilities of having it all. At the end of the day, I've learned to place the value on having what matters. The Old Testament gives us a great prompt in Proverbs 4:7 where it instructs that "wisdom is the principal thing [the most important thing]; therefore get wisdom: and with all thy getting get understanding [insight]." Thirty-eight years ago I stepped to purpose and began a journey to empower us in areas that I was seemingly unscripted for: journalism, television, public speaking. By faith, I showed up ready, and like David, who ran out to meet his opportunity in Goliath, I didn't shrink back. Without a journalism degree, without media training or courses in public speaking, just a tenacious desire to make a difference in every way imaginable, from looking the part on a dime to educating myself in the school of life, I began to represent us with honor as our First Lady of Beauty. What I know for sure today is that the King had a plan, and by faith I let him have his way. To this day it's a joy to get up every day no matter where I am in the world to go to work on our behalf. This calls for discipline, fortitude, and an unyielding determination to walk in the dreams of the ancestors who sacrificed that each of us might be free to be on purpose. Did it call for leading a prioritized life? Absolutely. As it does for many of us, it required me to set life in order because, as the

Word says, "To whom much is given, much is required." Of all the things life called for me to master, I knew I had to master Yours Truly first and foremost. So I set out to master "You Inc.," my court, from my internal sanctum to my temple, from my family to my palace, from honoring my purpose to the necessary management of human resources to see it through, and all the while remain focused on the vision because without vision, dreams are sure to vanish. Like any Queen balancing life, I know to this day that it calls for being resilient when the winds of adversity and negative influences come against me, and the ability to use them to catapult my growth. And finally, to use every waking moment to expand what is possible by giving my best.

66 I f best is possible, then good is not enough."
        —Chinese proverb

There are more adjectives to define life than I can say, but what's most important is this: it's *yours*, and you owe it to yourself to master it. How many of us are still looking for ourselves? Many of us have acquired identities not our own, and it shows in our lifestyle, in how we respond to others, in the way we dress and pursue our purpose, and in our lack of clarity concerning what's important to our joy and what's not. As I said at the beginning, life is not a dress rehearsal—this is it. When you fail to embrace your truth, in any area, for any reason whatsoever, how can you possess real joy? In order to master You Inc., you have to welcome the opportunity to do the internal work to be your authentic self because life is waiting for you to show up and have your say! To find yourself by releasing the clutter of all the stuff, both mentally and physically, so you can flourish. To be energized not by looking forward to the next promotion but by the brilliance you know exists within. The power of our thoughts can either move us forward and ensure an amazing life or hold us back from the joy we should embrace. It's time to recognize what we deserve and fill those shoes with gladness. We got this.

66 **T**ake responsibility for your actions, for the time you consume and for the space you occupy."

—Dr. Maya Angelou, poet, author, civil rights activist

These are no ordinary times, and in order to own the crown, you must be affirmed enough to refuse mediocrity and demonstrate the power you possess by example. To possess the courage to go for yourself and run full throttle in the direction of your dreams. When you do so, you inspire others to do the same, and as such, you become a force for change. It takes immeasurable faith to understand that the King has set you up to prosper in all and He will not fail. So don't settle for what shows up, He says. Ask for what you want and believe it's yours. So what does that look like in your life? What are your learns? What's your plan? To be effective, you must have a plan that's ready to activate. This is your opportunity, and in this diary I hope you have used those all-important "Notes to Self" pages to begin or refresh your strategy. Don't see them as resolutions or promises; be like the King and make a covenant with yourself by committing to this resolution with your signature:

I Am created for greatness

Born to succeed

Unique, unprecedented, and divine-inspired

I Am fully equipped, styled, fearfully and wondrously made

I Am called to transform, to lead and serve with gladness

I Am the evidence of dreams fulfilled

I Am love, joy, and purpose at work

I Will not give my power away, but use it to empower others

I Will render consistent execution in all things

Celebrating the truth of who I am with gratitude

Now go on and be the fine, fierce, and fearless Queen the King called you to be, and make it count. Master the art of being your divine self. Let your truism be like that of novelist Ayn Rand, whose edict was "The question isn't who's going to let me; it's who's going to stop me!"

Top 25 Takeaways to Master You Inc.

1. Take pride in being your authentic self and appreciate all that you are.

2. Don't eclipse your "it-ness." Celebrate your unique beauty and style sensibility with practices that affirm you without and within.

3. Be the gatekeeper to your mind. Don't give an all-access pass to that which will short-circuit your assurance, insult your intelligence, and destroy your courage to live out loud.

4. Create "time for self" to relax, refuel, and rejuvenate. You cannot serve and inspire from a place of lack.

5. "Self-care is not selfish; self-care is your responsibility to your future." —Lisa Nichols

6. Remember, any form of introspection is a valuable opportunity for renewal.

7. Be fearless, never shrink back, let your actions demonstrate that you know who you are.

8. You cannot be at peace if you are not centered in an identity that transcends the judgments of others or the circumstances that life brings your way.

9. Everything in your life stems from how you think and what you'll accept as fact, as well as the falsities that you allow to take up space in your mind and compromise your style.

10. Be sure you are nurturing what you want to grow and starving what you want to check.

11   Identify your gift (that divine assignment that you've been purposed to do) so you can lead and create.

12   You have the power to break the weight of the past. Do it so you can live fully in the present and affirm a clearer future.

13   Establish your celebration circle by identifying those who support you through thick and thin because supportive relationships promote your growth and keep you on purpose.

14   Challenge is where you have the capacity to grow the most, and you don't want to just "go through"; you want to grow through.

15   Cherish your beautiful brown skin like you would that of a newborn.

16   Real gratification that comes from investing in yourself is always worth the time. Pursue it.

17   It's not how beautiful your makeup is; it's how beautiful you are. That can't be purchased—don't lose sight of you!

18   "The key about makeup is looking like you were born with this skin." —Toni Acey

19   Prevent hair challenges. Put a plan in place that ensures healthy hair and styling practices that are well suited to maintaining it.

20   Great style begins within with an appreciation of who you are.

21   Don't get hung up on your dress size. Like age, it's just a number!

22   Stay on course. Maintain a clear, consistent style ID based on bankable, well-defined pieces.

23   Clear out the clutter, from the clothes you no longer wear to the things that confuse your distinction and diminish your mark.

24   Let go of your comfort zone so you can move into your power zone!

25   Remember, self-perception sets the tone for your life. Wake up every day excited to be you!

Notes to Self...

Notes to Self...

Acknowledgments

I Give Thanks . . .

To God, who makes all things possible, and my Lord and Savior Jesus Christ, through whom I have the ability to do all things.

For my mother, the late Modina Davis Watson, and my dad, Charles Graves, and the "Grands," whose wisdom continues to steer me on my journey.

For Taylor, my darling husband, in whose unconditional love I am hopelessly lost and forever found.

For the jewels in my crown, my children, Samantha, Philip Jr., and Ms. Ashley, of whom I couldn't be more proud.

For my Princess, Modina, the sweetest granddaughter in a million!

For my family, whose love I am more than blessed to have: my dear sister, Candace; my brother, Michael; my sister-in-love, Vandetta; brothers-in-love, Kenneth and Walter; and my gang—the cousins, nieces, and nephews.

For Pamela Macklin. Webster won't help me define my gratitude for the blessing that you are—love you, doll, forever!

For Sandra Martin, my "faith lamp," for your unwavering support, your sage advice, and your ability to make me believe I can do anything!

And for my celebration circle, and my brothers and sisters in Christ, and my colleagues, whose love and support makes all the difference in the journey.

And Praise . . .

To my literary agent, Claudia Menza, for the kind of encouragement that makes one fly!

To Judith Curr, publisher of Atria Books. It's so fabulous to be back "in the house"! Know that I'm honored by your support—you rock and I love you for it!

To my editors, Rakesh Satyal and Latoya Smith. Rakesh, for your priceless insights and patience while I worked without a clone! Thanks for convincing me that I had so much more to say. And Latoya, for your expertise and the joy you brought to the work.

To my executive coordinator, Jatika Hudson Patterson, for your dedication and coordination of the celebrity interviews for this project—know that I couldn't have done it without you.

To publicists, Joseph Babineaux and Nicole Newsum. You guys are a treasure!

To photographer Derek Blanks, for his visionary expertise and the ability to make every gal look fabulous!

To makeup artist Daryon Haylock, who brings the joy and wields a brush on a sitting like no other! Couldn't have sat for my closeup without you.

To Sheila Harris, my angel in the wings!

To the many experts whose time, vision, and brilliant insights will keep us all fabulously in the know! I bow.

About the Author

Mikki Taylor is the country's leading authority on "inner and outer beauty" for women of color, with more than thirty years of experience in media. Taylor is editor at large for *Essence* magazine and president of Satin Doll Productions, Inc., a strategic branding, consulting, and communications company. She is author of the critically acclaimed books *Self-Seduction* and *Commander in Chic*.